Healthful Publ
Stomach Ulcers: Symptoms, Solutions & Recipes
© 2020 Healthful Publications
info.healthful@gmail.com

This book is not intended as a substitute for the medical advice of physicians. The reader should regularly consult a physician in matters relating to his/her health, particularly with respect to any symptoms that may require diagnosis or medical attention. All readers are advised to seek medical and professional counsel before making any changes to their lifestyle and eating habits.

Table of Contents

Introduction

When we think of vital organs in the human body what comes to mind? The brain? The heart? The lungs? The gut is an extremely important part of the human physiology, and it hosts a forgotten organ, the gut microflora. Collectively, these tiny organisms contribute to our digestion, as well as aiding in nutrient absorption that fuels our journey throughout life. However, billions of people around the globe are suffering from disorders of the gut. Particularly common disorders include: Stomach Ulcers, Crohn's Disease, Irritable Bowel Syndrome, Small Intestinal Bacteria Overgrowth and Diverticulosis. The first description of a perforated ulcer dates back to 1670, England. Fast forward to modern times and its estimated that 4% of all adults above the age of 20 are currently experiencing an ulcer in either their stomach, small intestine, or both[1].

Stomach ulcers are not widely understood by the general public, and it's easy to understand why. There's even an air of confusion surrounding their very name. There are four distinct names depending on where they reside, here's a quick guide:

Location	Names
Stomach	Gastric/Peptic/Stomach Ulcer
Duodenum – first section of Small Intestine	Duodenal/Peptic/Stomach Ulcer

If you think you've noticed a mistake, you haven't. Ulcers within the stomach are called gastric ulcers. Those within the intestines are duodenal ulcers and the collective medical term for both are peptic ulcers. Peptic ulcer disease is the general term for those experiencing one or multiple peptic ulcers. Funnily enough, stomach ulcer is the most commonly used term for both forms of ulcer, primarily for simplicities sake since the symptoms and cure for both are the same. The remainder of this book will refer to ulcers as either stomach or peptic ulcers.

A peptic ulcer is defined as a wound in the lining of the stomach or intestinal wall that's greater than 3mm in diameter and with significant depth[2]. The most common form of ulcer is very shallow, carries minimal risk and causes minor discomfort. However, prolonged exposure to certain strains of bacteria as well as commonly taken medicine can exacerbate and increase the ulcers depth, ultimately causing complications. Not to worry, these causes are fully explained in the chapter "What Causes Stomach Ulcers?", and once aware of, are surprisingly easy to mitigate.

Symptoms of ulcers vary dramatically depending on their depth and location. On the mild spectrum, patients can experience pain after eating, either a few minutes or a few hours later; indigestion; heartburn; loss of appetite; vomiting or feeling nausea; and weight loss. More severe symptoms are indicators of ulcer complication and can include vomiting blood that may be bright red or dark brown similar to coffee grounds; passing dark, sticky stools; or a sudden, sharp pain in the abdomen that gets steadily worse. The symptoms and their causes are explained in the chapter "Symptoms Associated with Stomach Ulcers".

Unfortunately, there's been contradictory medical advice given to those that have had consultation before 1997 and those that received consultation after. It was previously believed that stress was the main cause of peptic ulcers, we now know this is not the case[3].

The consumption of various spices, caffeine and alcohol were also presumed to be a significant trigger in exacerbating or causing ulcers. This has also been debunked over time, instead playing an insignificant role[4]. In 1982, Dr Warren and Professor Marshall investigated the impact of a strain of bacteria by the name of Helicobacter Pylori (H. pylori) on gastritis (inflammation of the stomach lining) and peptic ulcer disease[5]. This discovery was so ground-breaking that it was previously believed impossible for any form of bacterium to be able to survive an environment so harsh as the gastric acid-filled stomach. How did Professor Marshall, a trainee doctor at the time, prove its link? The good old-fashioned way, by swallowing a culture of the bacterium and developing gastritis, which they diagnosed with an endoscopy and stomach biopsy[6]. It took until 1997 for the Center for Disease Control and Prevention, alongside government agencies and academic institutes to launch a national education campaign, teaching health care professionals and consumers the link between H. pylori and ulcers. In 2005 both Dr Warren and Professor Marshall were awarded a Nobel Prize in Physiology or Medicine for this discovery. We now know that the leading cause of gastric ulcers are H. Pylori and Nonsteroidal Anti-inflammatory Drugs (NSAIDs), which are discussed in detail in the sub-chapters "H. pylori" and "NSAIDs".

Fear not, it's not all doom and gloom. There are multiple medicinal and lifestyle choices available to either cure the disease or reduce symptoms to a point where an ulcer no longer impacts everyday life. This book thoroughly explores the exact nature of stomach ulcers; how they change your gastrointestinal physiology; which molecules and ingredients exacerbate ulcers; and which ones prevent further damage. The second half of this book contains 50 recipes specifically tailored to those with peptic ulcer disease. These recipes explain the precise benefits provided, such as whether this recipe contains a prebiotic effect that can reduce the density of H. pylori, as well as including their macronutrient content[28,30].

Our aim was to take the most complicated and thorough science from well-respected scientific papers, journals and studies, and translate their key messages into plain English. All quoted sources are fully referenced at the back of the book. Rest assured, none of the information in this book is obtained from non-scientific sources. The origins of these sources can be found by looking out for the small numbers at the end of sentences, taking this reference number and finding it in the "Sources" chapter. The reference will look like this:

[2] Yeomans, Neville D., and Jorgen Naesdal. "Systematic review: ulcer definition in NSAID ulcer prevention trials." *Alimentary pharmacology & therapeutics* 27, no. 6 (2008): 465-472.

It's not necessary to be able to read or understand scientific journals to read this book, but nevertheless, we have fully referenced them so they can be viewed at your curiosity. The example above can be broken down as follows:

- Reference Number = 2
- Authors = Yeomans, Neville D., and Jorgen Naesdal
- Title of Publication = "Systematic review: ulcer definition in NSAID ulcer prevention trials."
- Scientific Journal = Alimentary pharmacology & therapeutics 27, no. 6
- Year Published = (2008)
- Pages in Journal = 465-472

If you're interested in fully understanding the intricate details of how this disease changes the physiology of the patient, or simply how to maximize healing, read on!

How the Gut Works

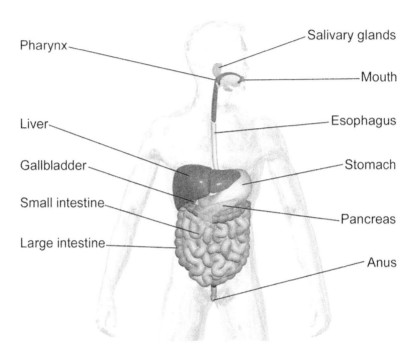

Figure 1 – The Digestive System. "Medical gallery of Blausen Medical 2014". WikiJournal of Medicine 1 (2). DOI:10.15347/wjm/2014.010. ISSN 2002-4436. Under Creative Commons BY (https://creativecommons.org/licenses/by/3.0), made greyscale

First things first, it's beneficial to gain a wider understanding of how the gut works in its entirety. If you're already well-versed in how the gut operates, feel free to skip this chapter.

The digestive system starts to work the moment food reaches your mouth and ends when it leaves your body. Food travels through a long tube with many twists and turns, being pushed through a series of processes that allow the body to absorb nutrients and remove waste. This tube is known by various names such as the alimentary canal, the gastrointestinal tract (GI tract/GIT), the digestive tract or the gut. The gut starts at the oral cavity (the mouth) and continues into the pharynx, esophagus, stomach, small intestine and finally the large intestine, which comprises of the cecum, colon, rectum and anal canal.

The process of digestion begins as soon as food enters the mouth. The food is broken into smaller particles and mixed with salivary enzymes when we chew. This concoction is then passed through the esophagus and into the stomach. The stomach introduces new enzymes and a highly acidic environment that breaks nutrients such as proteins, carbohydrates and fats into smaller sub-units such as peptides/amino acids, sugars, and lipids, respectively. These smaller sub-units are used to produce energy for our daily activities and contribute to our bodily maintenance. The stomach can also be used as a storage tank, allowing the rest of the gut to finish its digestive processes if the body has consumed a lot of food. The sub-units are then passed into the small intestine, which is where most of our nutrients are absorbed. Further enzymes from the pancreas and bile from the liver are then squeezed through ducts into the small intestine. The small intestine is made up of specialized cells that absorb nutrients as food passes through. These nutrients are then transferred into the bloodstream, where they are sent throughout the body to fuel various organs. The waste product is then passed into the large intestine, which absorbs any remaining nutrients and water before storing it in the rectum, awaiting mother nature's call.

There are many interlinked mechanisms that contribute to a healthy digestive system. Enzymes and acid break down food, tightly packed cells lining the small intestine precisely control the absorption of nutrients and a symbiotic army of bacteria patiently await their time to shine. The large intestine is home to this army, comprising of billions of beneficial micro-organisms that help digest the food we eat. You may have heard of these micro-organisms by their various aliases: microflora, microbiota, microbiome or simply, good gut bacteria. Some strains of bacteria are heavily relied upon to produce enzymes that break down carbohydrates the body cannot.

People suffering with digestive disorders can create a weak link in their digestive chain; impairing the body's ability to absorb nutrients, weakening many bodily functions; and upsetting the balance of their microflora ecosystem. If this intricate balance is disturbed, it can act as a catalyst for other diseases to occur. Similarly, if an underlying digestive disorder is fixed, it can grant multiple positive health benefits.

What Are Stomach and Duodenal Ulcers?

To recap: stomach ulcers are sometimes referred to as gastric ulcers; duodenum (first section of the small intestine) ulcers are referred to as duodenal ulcers; and peptic ulcer is a collective term for both. Despite the fact stomach ulcer literally refers to ulcers within the stomach, it's often used interchangeably for both types of ulcer as the symptoms and solutions of both are the same, even if the location is different. Peptic ulcers are defined as a lesion in the gastric or duodenal wall that's greater than 3mm in diameter and with significant depth[2]. An ulcers severity can be determined by how deeply it penetrates. If an ulcer penetrates deeply enough, it can erode a major blood vessel and potentially cause a life-threatening hemorrhage. Fortuitously, the most common form of ulcer is a mild erosion and carries minimal risks.

Peptic ulcers are caused by two main triggers: a bacterial infection called Helicobacter Pylori (H. pylori) and the use of NonSteroidal Anti-Inflammatory Drugs (NSAIDs) such as ibuprofen and aspirin. They can also be caused by minor lifestyle triggers such as smoking[7]. Unfortunately, peptic ulcer disease can occur in people of any age or gender. H. pylori is transmitted through food, water, utensils, saliva or bodily fluids and is frequently acquired as a child. A study in Germany on 1,806 people aged 18 to 89 years old concluded that 39.2% were H. pylori positive[8].

Those with peptic ulcer disease may experience no symptoms, acute symptoms or severe symptoms. Acute symptoms range from stomach pains to heartburn and even vomiting. Severe symptoms are caused from internal bleeding. Vomiting blood, passing dark, sticky stools or a sudden, sharp pain in the abdomen that gets steadily worse are categorized as severe symptoms and should be treated immediately by a physician.

In one of the largest studies of a general population to-date, a Swedish investigation found roughly 4% of 1,560 participants had a peptic ulcer[1]. The study included a varied group of people, all participants were over 20 years old, had a mean age of 50.4 years and 52% were male.

What Causes Stomach Ulcers?

Peptic ulcers are caused by excessive irritation to the walls of the stomach or first section of the small intestine, called the duodenum. A healthy human should possess multiple bodily mechanisms that serve as defensive measures against harm. One of these being mucus secretion, a barrier that protects the lining of the stomach and duodenum wall from stomach acid. Stomach acid is essential for breaking down food particles into the necessary nutrient components our bodies need to survive and grow. It is acidic by nature, which can become aggressive if not properly contained. Too little stomach acid can cause a lower absorption of nutrients, whereas too little mucus secretion can allow stomach acid to reach and irritate the wall lining. The body is exceptional at maintaining the balance between these aggressive and defensive forces. Unfortunately, this balance can be thrown off by external forces such as H. pylori and the use of NSAIDs.

If you're willing to learn the chemistry behind how stomach acid is produced and how the body prevents harm during each stage, feel free to flip to the sub-chapter "How Stomach Acid is Produced" in the "Appendix". Fair warning, we've tried to explain it as simply as possible whilst maintaining the juicy science, but it's still rather complex.

H. pylori

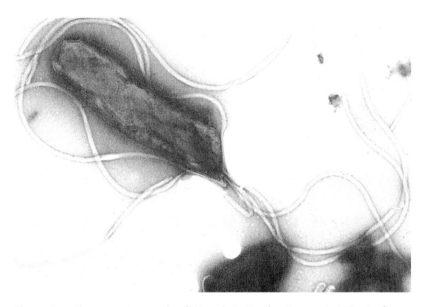

Figure 2 - Electron micrograph of H. pylori, Yutaka Tsutsumi, M.D. Professor, Department of Pathology Fujita Health University, School of Medicine / Copyrighted free use

H. pylori is a commonly occurring bacterium that's rampant throughout the world and is believed to thrive in food and water. People that reside in countries without access to clean water are at much higher risk of contracting this bacterium. However, it's impossible to completely prevent contact with H. pylori. The only known preventative technique is good hygiene, i.e. washing hands. A previously mentioned study of 1,806 people aged 18 to 89 years old concluded that 39.2% were H. pylori positive[8]. Irritation to the wall of the intestine or stomach is H. pylori's main offensive tactic, and it achieves this on multiple fronts.

H. pylori causes DNA methylation[9]. DNA methylation is the process of adding a methyl (CH$_3$) group to DNA, modifying it and affecting its function. Although this sounds scary, it's a common bodily function that's used to turn on and off DNA function where necessary. Without the ability to turn off DNA function, you wouldn't be able to stop many different automatic functions, such as producing mucus. Similarly, without the ability to turn on DNA function, your body wouldn't be able to start the healing process for internal abnormalities when they arise. The problem occurs when this methylation is caused unexpectedly by external forces. The DNA methylation that occurs from H. pylori in cells seems to disappear a few days after H. pylori is eradicated but will persist in stem-cells. A study published in 2019 accounts for 26 different genes that are affected by H. pylori[10]. The functions of these genes range from stabilizing the gastric mucus layer to enabling the process of autophagy (recycling cells that are no longer completely healthy). Therefore, H. pylori can reduce the defensive capability of the mucosal barrier as well as inhibiting the body's natural ability to heal stomach ulcers through DNA methylation.

H. pylori is a spiral shaped organism. Spiral shaped bacteria have been observed along the stomach wall, bypassing the thick layer of mucus that protects this wall from stomach acid[11]. It's theorized that this bacterium has evolved its spiral shape specifically to allow it to penetrate mucus[12]. Once H. pylori bypasses the mucus barrier, it goes on to colonize the stomach wall where it continually causes inflammation[13]. H. pylori that isn't able to reach the stomach wall have been observed to remain harmless, not causing any gastrointestinal problems[44].

One of the most cited meta-analysis regarding how H. Pylori and NSAIDs affect peptic ulcers was completed in 2002[14]. It states that a patient with H. pylori infection is 15.8% more likely to suffer from peptic ulcer disease than someone without H. pylori. They are also 6.3% more likely to have peptic ulcer bleeding.

NSAIDs

Nonsteroidal anti-inflammatory drugs (NSAIDs) are a family of drugs that reduce pain, decrease feverish temperatures and, as the name suggests, decrease inflammation. NSAIDs are some of the most prescribed group of drugs, and for good reason, they are lifesaving. The most common forms of NSAIDs are ibuprofen, naproxen and high-doses of aspirin (low-doses of aspirin are not normally considered a NSAID). Depending on the country of origin, these drugs may have different brand names, such as Ibuprofen being known as Advil in the United States, Ibalgin in the Czech Republic or Nurofen in multiple countries. Although NSAIDs are an excellent choice for combatting certain symptoms, by nature they are harsh on the gastrointestinal tract[15]. Their inherent acidity irritates the lining of the stomach wall whilst the same mechanism that dulls pain also reduces the production of a compound called prostaglandin. A reduction in prostaglandin causes an increase in gastric acid and decrease in mucus generation. Mucus is essential in protecting the lining of the stomach wall from gastric acid, making it especially harmful in large doses. In a 2004 drug safety study, they estimated that 38% of gastrointestinal bleeding have been caused by NSAIDs[16].

Back to the 2002 meta-analysis mentioned earlier[14]. NSAIDs are 27.5% more likely to cause uncomplicated peptic ulcer disease than not taking NSAIDs at all. They are also 32.3% more likely to cause peptic ulcer bleeding. In the presence of both a H. pylori infection and the use of NSAIDs, there's an increased risk of peptic ulcer disease by 3.55-fold.

Smoking

There is not enough empirical evidence to unanimously prove that smoking causes peptic ulcers, however, there is compelling evidence showing a correlation between smoking and peptic ulcer complication[17,18]. It's clear that those suffering with uncomplicated gastric ulcers have a much higher chance of complication if they smoke. In fact, smoking can increase chances of ulcer perforation 10-fold[19]. These results were similar whether in men or women, for gastric or duodenal ulcers. More specific studies have found that smoking by itself may not be a trigger, but smoking coupled with a H. pylori infection increases the chances greater than either of them individually[20].

Smoking causes numerous gastrointestinal changes to occur. Specifically, in relation to peptic ulcer disease, smoking causes: a reduction of circulating epidermal growth factor, which protects the mucosal barrier and heals stomach ulcers; modifies how blood flows through the gastric mucosa; disrupts angiogenesis, the formation of new blood vessels; and suppresses cell proliferation, the ability to create new cells which is essential for healing peptic ulcers[17]. Those that stopped smoking found no increase in risk.

Alcohol

Alcohol seems to have a minor effect on peptic ulcers, although this increases once coupled with other risk factors such as NSAIDs or H. pylori, its effects are significantly smaller than other factors[21].

Stress

Stress as a cause of peptic ulcer disease has fallen out of fashion since the discovery of H. pylori. Prior to this discovery, it was thought of as the biggest risk factor, which we now know to be incorrect. However, 10% of people with peptic ulcer disease have no sign of H. pylori and do not regularly take NSAIDs, meaning there are further risk factors that have not been fully identified[22]. Although it's hard to get empirical evidence on stress' direct link to peptic ulcer disease, there seems to be some unquantifiable connection. There's been an increased record of peptic ulcer disease following large disasters such as earthquakes, economic disasters and war[22]. Stress and its effects on healing have also been studied, mucosal wounds were given to dental students a few days before academic exams as well as during summer vacation, those given before exams took 40% longer to heal than those during vacation[23].

Spicy Food and Coffee

Once again, the previous hypothesis from the 20th century that spicy food and caffeine is a major risk factor for peptic ulcer disease has been debunked. The impact they have on existing ulcers are relatively minor, meaning that individuals are not required to exclude these from their diet, but can monitor individually whether they influence discomfort or not.

Summary

Peptic Ulcer Disease is often born from a combination of multiple risk factors, the most significant being H. pylori infection and frequent use of NSAIDs. If a patient tests positive for one major risk factor then minor risk factors, such as smoking and stress, play a much greater role in the possibility of contracting peptic ulcer disease.

Symptoms Associated with Stomach Ulcers

The symptoms of peptic ulcer disease can be categorized into 3 stages: uncomplicated (no symptoms), acute symptoms and severe symptoms. Uncomplicated patients are more likely to have an ulcer that is either too small in diameter or depth to cause any issues, but the patient should be mindful not to aggravate the ulcer. A patient suffering from acute symptoms may experience stomach pain that can travel from the middle of the abdomen up to the neck and back down to either the belly button or back[24]. This pain normally starts after eating and can start after a few minutes or even a few hours, sometimes during the night. Antacids (medication that neutralizes stomach acid) may temporarily relieve the pain, but it won't cure the ulcer. Other acute symptoms are indigestion; heartburn; loss of appetite; vomiting or feeling nausea; and weight loss.

Those suffering severe symptoms should contact their doctor immediately or call emergency services. Severe symptoms include vomiting blood that may be bright red or dark brown similar to coffee grounds; passing dark, sticky stools; or a sudden, sharp pain in the abdomen that gets steadily worse. Severe symptoms are markers that indicate more dangerous complications.

The most common complication is when an ulcer develops at the site of a blood vessel, causing internal bleeding[24]. Severe bleeding will cause black, sticky stools or vomiting blood. Slow, long-term bleeding causes fatigue, breathlessness, pale skin and heart palpitations. If the patient is suffering from severe blood loss, a surgeon may have to perform an endoscopy to identify the cause and location as well as performing a surgical procedure to repair the site of damage and affected blood vessel. Blood transfusions may also be delivered to replace lost blood.

Perforation of the stomach (stomach lining splitting open), is a rare complication that can cause bacteria from the stomach to infect the lining of the abdomen. This is called peritonitis and is life threatening if left untreated. Peritonitis requires hospital admission which can last up to 14 days. Antibiotics will be administered directly into the vein (intravenously). If the stomach lining is damaged or infected, surgery may be required to repair the damaged site and any pus-filled swellings may need to be drained.

Gastric outlet obstruction occurs when the stomach ulcer blocks the passage of food through the digestive system. This can cause repeated vomiting that contains undigested food; persistent bloating; feeling very full after eating a small amount of food; and unexplained weight loss. Obstructions are usually caused by two bodily mechanisms: inflammation or scar tissue. It takes a reduction in stomach acid to create a less acidic environment that allows swelling to reduce and inflammation to decrease. This is achieved by prescription of either a proton pump inhibitor or H2-receptor antagonist, which are described fully in the chapter "How to Heal Stomach Ulcers". If the obstruction is caused by scar tissue, a surgeon may need to operate, however, sometimes a small balloon can be passed through the obstruction and inflated to widen the site without surgery.

Thankfully, most peptic ulcers remain uncomplicated. By seeking professional diagnosis before an ulcer reaches its more severe stages, it's possible to mitigate life-threatening risks.

Diagnosing Stomach Ulcers

The first step in treating a disorder is correctly identifying it, which is why professional diagnosis is a necessity. Many gastrointestinal disorders share similar symptoms making an incorrect diagnosis, especially a self-diagnosis, a possibility. An incorrect diagnosis could mean using false treatments that do not work at all, alleviate the symptoms but not the underlying disease or make the disorder worse. Gastrointestinal disorders that share similar symptoms with peptic ulcers include indigestion; irritable bowel syndrome; diverticular disease; appendicitis; kidney stones; inflammatory bowel disease such as Crohns disease or ulcerative colitis; gastritis or even bowel, pancreatic and stomach cancer.

If a patient is experiencing any peptic ulcer-like symptoms and visits a doctor, they will most likely be tested for H. pylori infection via a breath test, since it's minimally invasive. This breath test consists of breathing into a device, drinking warm water mixed with a urea compound and then breathing once again into the device[25]. H. pylori digests this urea compound and produces isotope-labelled carbon dioxide which the breath test can pick up. If no H. pylori is present, the compound will naturally be eradicated. Alternative methods of detecting H. pylori include a fecal (aka stool test) or serology test (aka blood test). The fecal test looks for foreign proteins produced by H. pylori that aren't naturally produced by the body, these foreign proteins are called antigens. Serum is a component of blood and includes all proteins not used in blood clotting; all electrolytes, antigens, antibodies, hormones; and any exogenous substances (e.g., drugs or microorganisms). Serum is also used as a term for any fluid that resembles serum, such as the fluid in a blister. A serology test analyses the serum for antibodies produced by H. pylori. These antibodies continue to inhabit the bloodstream even after H. pylori has been eradicated, so if the patient has previously taken specific forms of antibiotics this test may return a false positive.

The most precise methods of detecting peptic ulcer disease are more invasive and require analysis of gastrointestinal tissue. Aside from the H. pylori breath test, a physician might request a Barium Swallow, Endoscopy or Endoscopic Biopsy. A Barium swallow is a procedure in which the patient drinks a thick white liquid called barium, this liquid coats the upper gastrointestinal tract and allows doctors a more detailed view of the stomach and small intestine via X-ray.

An endoscopy involves inserting an endoscope, a thin tube with a camera, through the mouth and into the stomach and small intestine to check for ulcers or abnormal tissue. An endoscopic biopsy is the most invasive but is the most accurate in terms of differentiating between various diseases simultaneously. An endoscope that's equipped with a surgical tool is passed through to the affected tissue, a small amount is then removed and analyzed in a lab. In 1964 the first endoscope equipped with a camera was invented. With the dramatic advancements in technology since then, particularly in computer chips and image processing, modern day endoscopes are incredibly powerful and much easier to use[26]. With our access to newer medical devices as well as our collectively greater understanding of peptic ulcers, doctors and gastroenterologists have a much higher chance of successful diagnosis than ever before.

How to Heal Stomach Ulcers

A two-pronged attack is required to eliminate the root cause of peptic ulcer disease as well as creating the optimal healing environment. We are now well aware that peptic ulcers are caused by two major triggers, H. pylori and NSAIDs, as well as a handful of minor triggers which become serious once multiple are combined.

Temporary Symptom Relief

Proper treatment may take an entire day to relieve the immediate pain caused by an ulcer. Your doctor may prescribe antacids and alginates to neutralize stomach acid and create a protective coating on the lining of the stomach, respectively. These should be taken as prescribed and assist with temporarily reducing stomach pain.

Addressing the Root Cause

H. Pylori

H. pylori is a bacterial infection and as with all bacterial infections, antibiotics are the most effective method of eradication. A physician will most likely prescribe either a single antibiotic, or multiple to be taken in conjunction. Common prescriptions being amoxicillin, clarithromycin or metronidazole for two weeks, twice a day, although you should follow your physician's direct recommendation. It's important to take the full course as directed by a physician, as taking a shorter course may temporarily cure the symptoms but allow stronger strains of bacteria to survive, which may cause reinfection that is harder to cure later down the road[27]. In fact, antibiotic treatment for H. pylori is only 90% effective due to its growing antibiotic resistance[28]. A systematic review of H. pylori antibiotic resistance in 2010 found the resistance rates were: 17.2% for clarithromycin, 26.7% for metronidazole, 11.2% for amoxycillin, 16.2% for levofloxacin, 5.9% for tetracycline, 1.4% for rifabutin and 9.6% for multiple antibiotics[29].

Probiotic (foods or supplements rich with live, healthy bacteria and yeasts) treatment taken in conjunction with antibiotics may alleviate negative side-effects such as diarrhea, taste disturbance, vomiting and nausea[28]. If your physician prescribes you antibiotics, then feel free to ask which probiotics they recommend. In a 7 study meta-analysis, overall, patients that took probiotics alongside antibiotics had a 20% chance of incurring less side-effects than those taking antibiotics only[28]. It's important to mention that taking probiotics did not eradicate H. pylori alone, nor did it increase the effectiveness of eradicating H. pylori in this meta-analysis. There is, however, evidence that probiotics reduces H. pylori density in animals and humans, particularly the probiotic lactobacilli[30]. A lower density potentially means that the negative effects of H. pylori infection are similarly reduced. A systematic review of 16 studies that assessed the impact of probiotics on H. pylori confirmed the meta-analysis' finding above. Probiotics do not eradicate H. pylori but there's evidence to suggest that they decrease H. pylori density, decrease side-effects of antibiotics and increase defensive mechanisms such as stabilizing the gastric barrier function and decreasing mucosal inflammation[31].

Vitamin C (Cabbage Juice)

Before the discovery of H. pylori, a popular natural remedy for peptic ulcer disease was the humble cabbage juice. This remedy has understandably fallen out of fashion for two reasons: the rise of modern medicine and the lack of evidence proving how cabbage juice promotes ulcer healing. However, there are interesting recent studies indicating why cabbage juice may in fact be beneficial.

Fresh cabbage is high in Vitamin C, a 10.5oz (300g) portion equates to 110mg of Vitamin C, or 122% of the recommended daily intake. 10.5oz (300g) is extremely hard to eat alone, however, juicing it makes this challenge infinitely easier. A study in 1998 tested Vitamin C's effects on 60 patients with H. pylori related inflammation of the stomach (gastritis)[32]. It found that 4 weeks of daily high dose vitamin C treatment resulted in the eradication of H. pylori in 30% of those treated as well as a high concentration of Vitamin C in their stomach acid which continued for 4 weeks post-study. They were not able to observe negative effects from high doses of Vitamin C. It's not recommended to consume more than 2000mg of Vitamin C daily, although this would require consuming 142 oranges. However, they were not able to link why or how Vitamin C effects H. pylori, so further research is required. Another study in 1997 conducted by a department of infectious disease and tropical medicine by a Tokyo based department research institute also investigated this hypothesized link[33]. They found that vitamin C could inhibit the growth of 90% of bacterial strains, even those incubated in slightly acidic environments, similar to that of the mucosal barrier where H. pylori resides. Once again, however, the method in which Vitamin C impacts H. pylori is unknown.

NSAIDs

If you regularly take ibuprofen, naproxen, aspirin or other NSAIDs then you should inform your physician immediately and they will help transition you to alternative forms of medication. Paracetamol is widely considered a safer alternative to ibuprofen. In a twelve-study systematic review conducted in Spain in 2005, the researchers concluded the most commonly used doses of paracetamol conferred little or no increased risk of gastrointestinal complication[34]. Daily low-dose aspirin is sometimes prescribed as a blood thinning medication to prevent heart attacks, strokes and blood clots. Your doctor will advise on whether it's safer to continue taking aspirin as it's considered to be an NSAID when taken in high doses.

Allowing Ulcers to Heal

The body is equipped to automatically find and heal certain types of gastrointestinal disorders, peptic ulcers being one of them. The body is host to a wide range of intricate mechanisms that are essential for repair and growth. Sometimes these beneficial mechanisms become harmful when the body's natural order is disrupted. One excellent example being stomach acid. Stomach acid is essential for extracting nutrients from food but is also irritating to peptic ulcers and can prevent healing, or in severe circumstances, cause perforation. We'll look at the bodies automatic healing response, how smoking alters this physiological response, artificially reducing gastric acid and an interesting supplement by the name of Zinc-Carnosine.

Physiological Healing Mechanisms

Ulcers are genetically programmed to be healed by the body via a series of mechanisms consisting of cell migration, cell proliferation, re-epithelialization, formation of granulation tissue, angiogenesis and tissue remodeling[35]. All of these processes are stimulated by cytokines and growth factors. Although this might sound extremely confusing, their mechanisms are simple to explain at a high-level overview.

Epidermal Growth Factor (EGF) is a protein produced by cells and the salivary gland. EGF plays multiple roles; it moves from cell to cell and controls the cells ability to grow and multiply; it searches for an EGF receptor to bind to, which stimulates a chain of biochemical healing reactions; and plays a part in mucosal protection from gastric acid[36]. Once EGF is bound to an EGF receptor the following begins, not necessarily in order:

- Glycolysis - the breakdown of glucose into various molecules such as adenosine triphosphate (ATP) that provides energy to cells.
- Protein synthesis - proteins are created. Proteins are used in multiple healing processes within the body.
- DNA synthesis - creation of DNA.
- Specific gene expression increases - information from a gene is used to create something, often proteins.
- Cell proliferation - a total increase in cells that starts with cells growing in size and then dividing into two separate cells.
- Cell migration - as the name suggests, the movement of cells to specific locations in the body.
- Re-epithelialization - a barrier like function that makes cells cover an injured site in a scar.
- Granulation tissue creation - connective tissue created at the base of a wound that will eventually fill the entire wound with new tissue and blood vessels.
- Angiogenesis - the creation of new blood cells.
- Tissue remodeling - this is the final phase of wound healing and is complete once the wound is fully filled with new tissue and blood vessels.

Those high-level summaries make it clear how many complex steps are involved in the healing of ulcers. Any disruption can inhibit the healing process, which can aggravate ulcers and cause serious complications.

Implications of Smoking

Although there's not conclusive evidence to suggest smoking directly causes peptic ulcer disease, there's plenty of evidence to suggest that it reduces the body's natural ability to heal from ulcers and other gastrointestinal problems.

A 1992 study followed 10 smokers that smoke 20 or more cigarettes per day for at least 5 years as well as 5 non-smokers. It found that the smokers produce 32% less Salivary Epidermal Growth Factor (EGF) than the non-smokers[37]. As we know from above, EGF plays a vital role in starting the chain of ulcer healing mechanisms. Heavy smoking reduces EGF which suppresses angiogenesis and cell proliferation . This is not to be confused with cancer, which is unique in its ability to abnormally proliferate, bypassing the precise regulation that EGF controls and spreading throughout the body unchecked[38]. Smoking also reduces mucus secretion, the mucus barrier is a potent defense mechanism that stops gastric acid from touching the stomach wall.

Proton Pump Inhibitors

To greatly reduce the amount of gastric acid generated, your physician will most likely prescribe a proton pump inhibitor (PPI) for 4-8 weeks, the most commonly recommended being omeprazole, pantoprazole or lansoprazole. A PPI is, as the name suggests, a drug that inhibits (stops) the proton pump which is responsible for pushing H^+ into the stomach in exchange for K^+. Without H^+, Cl^- can't combine to create HCl (hydrochloric acid). The chemical reaction is fully explained in the

Appendix, sub-chapter "How Stomach Acid is Produced". PPIs are able to reduce up to 99% of acid secretion in this manner and allow ulcers to heal in a non-acidic environment. Ulcers take roughly 4-8 weeks to heal, which is why the prescribed course is typically 4-8 weeks.

H$_2$ Receptor Antagonists

Your physician might also prescribe a H$_2$ receptor antagonist. Although not as effective as PPIs, they also reduce gastric acid secretion. The parietal cell contains receptors that, once stimulated, produce gastric acid. H$_2$ receptor antagonists then, as the name suggests, blocks this receptor and reduces the amount of gastric acid that the parietal cells can produce.

Natural Methods of Reducing Acid

There have been numerous tests and studies investigating everything from prolonged fasting to specific diets, such as the elemental diet[39]. However, unless your physician recommends you adopt an additional method of gastric acid reduction, you should refrain from doing so. This is due to Proton Pump Inhibitors and H$_2$-Receptor Antagonists extreme efficacy at reducing gastric acid, making alternative methods redundant if not harmful. Not only can acid reduction be properly controlled and timed using these medications, gastric acid is essential for breaking down food, killing bacteria and providing nutrition, which means attempts to further reduce gastric acid may negatively impact health. Luckily for us, there are alternative and safer methods of promoting gastric healing which are discussed in the chapter "Ingredient Analysis".

Alternative Remedies for Stomach Ulcers

This section contains details about a very intricate three-part scientific study and has been kept as close so the source material as possible. Due to this, it's quite science-heavy, however, it gives you a behind-the-scenes look at something the everyday person doesn't see. If things are too confusing, fear not, have a look at each table and then skip to the last paragraph that summarizes the entire study.

There are many foods that contain Zinc, Carnosine or both, such as meat, fish and dairy. The magic happens once both molecules are combined artificially, providing benefits much stronger than the sum of their parts. Zinc-carnosine (ZnC) is an artificially produced health supplement that's created by combining a zinc ion and carnosine in a 1-to-1 ratio. ZnC can be bought in many health shops under different brand names such as Pepzin GI, as well as a commonly prescribed tablet called Polaprezinc in Japan for treating peptic ulcers. Although relatively unknown in the western world, the gastrointestinal healing effects of ZnC have been well studied. A comprehensive study comprised of three separate tests were conducted in England and found very intriguing results[40].

The first test investigated the effects of ZnC on intestinal permeability, that is, the cells ability to stop material passing through it, such as stopping molecules from passing through the cells lining the gut wall and keeping them in the gastrointestinal tract. A common technique for assessing intestinal permeability is known as the lactulose-rhamnose intestinal permeability test. This test involves patients emptying their bladders after an overnight fast and then drinking a sugar solution that consists of three different molecular-sized sugars. Urine is collected over the next five hours and analyzed for its lactulose:rhamnose ratio (L:R). Lactulose is a larger molecule than rhamnose, meaning that it cannot freely pass through the intestinal wall into the urine, whilst rhamnose can. Therefore, those suffering with high intestinal permeability will have higher L:R ratios than those that do not.

Ten healthy volunteers that were not taking NSAIDs and had no previous reason for increased intestinal permeability were tested. Each morning they were given this lactulose-rhamnose solution, their urine was then collected over the next five hours and their L:R was analyzed. Here's a quick summary:

Part	Routine	Mean L:R Ratio after 7 days
1	2 days ZnC, additional 5 days ZnC & Indomethacin	0.3
Two Week Break to Reset Participants Systems		
2	2 days Placebo, additional 5 days Placebo & Indomethacin	0.9

Table 1 – First Study, Intestinal Permeability effects of ZnC. ZnC successfully reduced the L:R by 3-fold compared to the control.

For the first half of the study, they were given ZnC for two days, then ZnC and the NSAID indomethacin for 5 more days. NSAIDs are known to cause intestinal permeability. The patients L:R remained consistent in the entire first section of the study, even after the last 5 days of taking indomethacin alongside ZnC. The participants took a two-week break to flush their systems before the next stage. After the break, they were then given a placebo for two days, then the placebo and indomethacin for the next 5 days. Their L:R were three-times higher at the end of the placebo testing stage compared to the ZnC testing stage. Therefore, indomethacin increased intestinal permeability, allowing the larger lactulose molecules to seep through whilst ZnC prevented it. This demonstrates ZnC's potent ability at combatting intestinal permeability.

The second study involved testing the direct effect ZnC has on ulcer healing in rats. Here's a quick summary:

Drug	Mean % Reduction in Gastric Injury 3 hours post-Indomethacin, Compared to Placebo
EGF	84%
ZnC	75%

Table 2 – Second Study, % Reduction in Gastric Injury from ZnC. ZnC showed similar gastric injury prevention qualities to EGF.

These rats were given either a placebo, ZnC or Epidermal Growth Factor (EGF), then after 30 minutes they were given indomethacin and left for a further 3 hours. As we've already discussed, EGF is a potent protein that places a leading role in starting natural ulcer healing mechanisms. At the end of the study, the rats were killed and the placebo, ZnC and EGF fed rats were analyzed for gastrointestinal damage. The rats fed ZnC had a 75% reduction in gastric injury compared to those that received the placebo. The results showed a similar reduction of gastric injury in those that received EGF and those receiving ZnC.

The final study was split into two parts, investigating how ZnC affects both cell migration and cell proliferation. Both parts were achieved by placing cells in petri dishes, "wounding" them by scraping a pipette tip across the dish and then treating them with either ZnC, Zinc Sulphate or Bovine Serum Albumin (BSA). Here's a quick summary:

Solution	Cell Migration (% Increase vs. Baseline)	Cell Proliferation (^{3}H Thymidine incorporation (cpm x 10^3))
BSA (Control)	No Significant Effect	11
Zinc Sulphate	No Significant Effect	19
ZnC	300%	40.5

Table 3 – Third Study, ZnC's effect on Cell Migration and Cell Proliferation levels in human cells.

Cell migration was tested by taking periodic microscopic images and monitoring how far cells move after the "wounding". ZnC caused a 3-fold increase in the distance cells migrated from their baseline. Cell proliferation was tested by adding ^{3}H Thymidine (which is radioactive and easy to detect) to different quantities of ZnC, Zinc Sulphate and Bovine Serum Albumin. Newly created (proliferated) cells incorporate the radioactive material into their DNA, which can be measured, allowing scientists the ability to analyze the rate of cell multiplication. The ZnC fed petri dishes had two-times the incorporation than the Zinc Sulphate dishes, and four-times than the Bovine Serum Albumin dishes.

In summary, this study showed that ZnC had positive effects on intestinal permeability, reducing gastric injury and improving two healing mechanisms: cell migration and cell proliferation. Intestinal permeability, or the cells ability to stop material passing through it and keeping material where they should be, was shown to be increased 3-fold in subjects taking ZnC compared to a placebo. Gastric injury was reduced by 75% in rats that were fed ZnC compared to a placebo. Cell migration was increased by 3-fold compared to baseline and cell proliferation 4-fold compared to the control. A few other interesting notes arose from this study. ZnC only influenced growth on cells with damage, meaning there is no positive benefit of taking ZnC for people without ulcers or other forms of gastrointestinal damage. The ZnC used in these studies correlate similarly to quantities that can be found in food supplements.

Recent Advancements in Science

On a daily basis, science pushes the limits of our understanding to new heights. This makes it hard, if not impossible, for everyone but gastroenterologists and those dedicated to specific medical niches to maintain the most up-to-date knowledge. However, it's important to note that new information doesn't automatically qualify it as superior information. The most reliable studies are those that have been well established and included in wide-ranging meta-analyses/systematic reviews or have been used as a basis for further investigation. Although it never hurts to stay one step ahead. Below are some interesting avenues that have been discovered lately but proceed with a skeptical mind until other researchers have had time to investigate their claims. Interestingly, a significant amount of research is being published regarding pushing the boundaries of Dr Warren and Professor Marshall's Nobel prize winning H. pylori discovery conducted in 1982.

The Spiral Shape of H. Pylori and Its Potential Treatment

H. pylori can penetrate the stomachs mucosal barrier by twisting its spiral shape like a screw piercing wood[41]. Its shape alone is an integral mechanism that allows it to be so disruptive. A study done by Fed Hutchinson Cancer Research Center in 2020 found that two specific proteins, MreB and CcmA, are responsible for balancing both sides of H. pylori's cell-wall production, forming its spiral shape. Further studies are required to investigate if these proteins can be eradicated, and if this is observed to stop H. pylori from maintaining its spiral shape. Further studies are then required to prove if H. pylori without this shape is unable to properly reach the mucosal barrier and infect the host. If all of this is true, then essentially, this lays out the potential for specific antibiotics or other forms of medicine that can target these proteins. They could have a less destructive impact on healthy bacteria, reducing negative side-effects whilst maintaining ulcer healing efficacy.

H. Pylori and Its Relation to Neurological Treatment

A systematic review done by the Journal of Parkinson's disease discovered some interesting findings[42]. Parkinson's disease sufferers were 1.5 to 3 times more likely to be infected with H. pylori than people without Parkinson's. H. pylori infected Parkinson's disease patients displayed worse motor functions that those without H. pylori. Once H. pylori was eradicated, the patients gained improved motor function. The eradication of H. pylori was met with an increased levodopa absorption, levodopa being an important amino acid that helps regulate dopamine amongst other molecules and is often prescribed as a supplement to Parkinson's disease patients, reducing the intensity of their symptoms. Interestingly, Parkinson's disease is often preceded by gastrointestinal dysfunction, which means that this condition could originate from the gut and spread to the brain along the brain-gut axis, which has been documented in rats[43]. It's more likely that this is one small part of a much larger puzzle, which is promising but needs to be investigated at much greater length.

H. Pylori Isn't All Bad

It seems like H. Pylori is nothing but trouble, hellbent on causing problems for its host. This isn't true in all cases, in fact, only 10% of people that are infected with H. pylori also suffer from some form of gastrointestinal disease. There is even evidence demonstrating H.

pylori can protect against esophageal cancer and asthma in the right environments[44]. A study led by scientists at the University of California found that genetically identical mice, whose origins came from two different suppliers, had two different responses to H. pylori[45]. Even though these mice were genetically identical, they had differences in their gastrointestinal microflora. Mice that contracted H. pylori but showed no signs of inflammatory disease had more than 4,000 differences in gut bacteria composition or concentrations compared to the mice that did have inflammatory disease. Although they couldn't conclusively state which species impedes the negative effects of H. pylori, there is one indication that points towards the Clostridium species, however, more research is needed. This paves way for potentially treating H. pylori with probiotics instead of antibiotics once the correct strains and quantities are fully verified.

Sleep Quality's Impact on Peptic Ulcer Recurrence

A Chinese study published in 2019 followed 1,420 Chinese patients that received anti-ulcer treatment and had successfully recovered from peptic ulcer disease[46]. They tracked these patients for up to 36 months via questionnaires and various sleep tracking devices. Unfortunately, 2.8% of these patients had a recurrence of peptic ulcer disease per year. This is one of the only studies on this subject matter and needs to be thoroughly counter studied, so take these results with a grain of salt. They found that patients that reported bad sleep quality had a 1.895-times likelihood of ulcer recurrence than those that reported good sleep quality. Based on results received from their sleep test equipment, they found patients were 69% more likely to have ulcer recurrence if they had a greater number of awakenings than those that did not and 55% more likely if they took longer to fall asleep compared to those that fell asleep quicker. Longer total sleep time seemed to prevent ulcer recurrence, reducing the likelihood of another ulcer appearing by 23% compared to those that acquired less sleep. However, many of the patients also suffered from other diseases: such as cardiovascular, diabetes or mental illness. Some of the patients also reported excessive alcohol consumption. Although interesting, it's hard to triangulate which specific factors caused a reduction in ulcer recurrence. However, this could lead to more research investigating the direct effect on ulcer recurrence related to activities that increase sleep quality, such as regular exercise, lower alcohol consumption and mental health support.

Ingredient Analysis

Since traditional anti-ulcer treatment has an 82.4% success rate, few physicians recommend other methods of treatment[47]. The causes of peptic ulcers are unanimously concrete, and medicinal treatments are well established. There are also engrained healing mechanisms observed within the body that can be promoted with certain molecules, vitamins and minerals. What if the promotion of these mechanisms could improve daily life? This chapter analyses all manners of food in search of the highest concentrations and cheapest sources of these molecules. It's important to note that the methods laid out are not to be used as a substitute for professional treatment.

Mucus Production

The formation of peptic ulcers is due to an imbalance between aggressive factors, such as the use of NSAIDs, and defensive factors, such as mucus production[48]. Some aggressive factors also decrease the effectiveness of defensive factors, such as NSAIDs ability to reduce mucus production as well as increase stomach acid production. There are no routinely prescribed drugs targeted towards increasing the body's natural defense mechanisms. There is, however, plenty of evidence citing the direct link increased mucus production has on the reduction of peptic ulcer formation, as well as which molecules increase mucus production[48].

As has already been discussed, the Mucosal-bicarbonate barrier is an integral defense mechanism that protects the stomach lining from stomach acid. Fiber in oat bran, rye bran and soybean hull have shown to increase goblet cell volume density (mucosal goblet cells being responsible for secreting mucus). Short chain fatty acids (most notably butyrate) directly stimulate mucus production as well as certain probiotics possessing a short-term stimulating effect[49].

Butyrate (aka butyric acid) is currently the most promising short-chain fatty acid as it seems to be the most effective in stimulating mucus release[50]. Butyrate has been observed to modulate mucin gene expression in goblet cells, this gene expression spurs the goblet cells to release mucus by up to 1.6-times the normal amount[51]. Although there are traces of Butyrate in animal fat, plant oils and animal milk, the highest concentrations of butyrate are produced by the fermentation of dietary fiber by healthy gut bacteria. Butyrate is a primary source of energy for multiple types of cells, particularly those in the large intestine and helps regulate their function[52]. Therefore, dietary fiber (probiotics) and prebiotic rich foods can play a positive role in improving the body's natural ulcer defense mechanisms.

Reducing H. Pylori

Probiotics help combat the negative side-effects of antibiotics as well as reducing the density of H. pylori[28,30]. For a more detailed explanation, feel free to revisit the sub-chapter "Addressing the Root Cause" in the chapter "How to Heal Stomach Ulcers". This makes promoting the density and variety of healthy bacteria extremely beneficial. A highly diverse intestinal flora contributes to general digestive wellbeing and assists with all manners of digestion[53,54]. There are two dietary methods for increasing intestinal flora count; consuming foods rich with live bacteria and yeasts (aka probiotics) or consuming foods that gut microflora consume themselves (aka prebiotics) such as the fibrous foods mentioned above.

As mentioned previously, foods high in Vitamin C have also been shown to reduce levels of H. pylori. The previous study found that 4 weeks of daily high dose vitamin C treatment resulted in the eradication of H. pylori in 30% of those treated and a continued high concentration of Vitamin C concentration in their stomach acid for 4 weeks after the study[32].

Summary

The two main ulcer treatments are reducing stomach acid from contacting any existing ulcers and reducing the efficacy of H. pylori. It's possible to compliment these goals by consuming certain molecules that increase mucus production and lower H. pylori density. Although it's not possible to cure stomach ulcers by diet alone, there is evidence that shows certain dietary changes can improve the efficacy of traditional medicinal treatment. Fibrous fermentable foods boost mucus production, probiotics stimulate mucus production, and probiotics alongside Vitamin C help lower the density of H. pylori.

High Fiber Foods

If you're already well versed in the several types of Fiber, feel free to skip the next paragraph.

First off, carbohydrates have three sub-classifications, sugars, starch and fiber. Some foods high in carbohydrates have little fiber, such as white bread and white rice. There's a tremendous amount of confusion over the definitions of various forms of fiber, especially on the internet. The term Dietary Fiber simply means fiber that is readily available through food, whereas Functional Fiber is the term for fiber that is synthetically added to processed food and is either extracted from natural food sources or manufactured. Three characteristics can describe fiber: solubility, viscosity and fermentability. The most common classification being solubility: either soluble or insoluble. Insoluble fiber doesn't break down in water whereas soluble fiber does. Soluble fibers are also known as prebiotics because of their direct beneficial impact on healthy gut bacteria, which the next sub-chapter focuses exclusively on. Viscosity is the fibers ability to thicken in the presence of water, very viscous fibers can form a gel in the presence of water which is why it's possible to make fruit jams. Fermentability determines if the fiber can be readily digested by the gut microflora, which they break down into short-chain fatty acids like the aforementioned butyrate.

Unfortunately, the beneficial effects of certain types of fiber where discovered fairly recently. For example, all insoluble fiber was considered to have no beneficial effect on the gut microflora and was primarily used to create soft and easier-to-pass stool. We now know that specific types of insoluble fiber, termed resistant starch, are resistant to the digestive process. This resistant starch passes through the stomach, small intestine and into the large intestine: which is where it can feed the largest colony of gut bacteria. Luckily for us, foods that are rich in non-fermentable fiber also contain fiber that is fermentable, so it's not necessary to micromanage the consumption of specific types of fiber. For the purpose of producing the most Butyrate, this section will look at natural foods highest in total fiber.

Fermentability	Examples of Fiber
Fermentable	Beta-Glucans, Gums, Inulin, Hemicelluloses, Resistant Starches, Pectin & Oligofructose
Poorly Fermented	Cellulose & Lignin

Grains

As a general rule, all grains, especially wholegrains, are high in fiber. Wholegrain simply means that the entirety of the grain is left intact, essentially the grain is left as it was growing in the field. Advancement in milling technology allowed the bran and germ to be removed cheaply and easily, turning wholegrains such as brown rice into a refined version, white rice. The center part of the grain, endosperm, is considered the most flavorful and is easier to cook than the wholegrain. However, we are now aware that 70% of the nutrients come from the other two parts of the grain, the bran and germ. There is also a lot more fiber in wholegrain than refined grain, for example, whole wheat flour contains 4-5x more fiber than white flour.

High Fiber Grains

Food	Fiber per cup	Fiber per 100 grams	Cost
Oats	16.5	10.6	$
Buckwheat	17	10	$$
Wholegrain Cornmeal	8.9	7.3	$
Whole-wheat Bread (per slice)	1.9	6	$
Bulgur	8.2	4.5	$
Whole-wheat Pasta	4.5	3.9	$
Quinoa	5.2	2.8	$$
Brown Rice	3.5	1.8	$
Couscous	2.2	1.4	$$
Egg Noodles	1.9	1.2	$
Rice Noodles	1.8	1	$

Low Fiber Grains for Comparison

Food	Fiber per cup	Fiber per 100 grams
White Pasta	3.7	3.2
White Bread	0.8 per slice	2.7
White Rice	0.6	0.4

Fruits

Most fruit are high in fiber if their skin is kept intact. Prices for the same fruit vary depending on season. Not only is it much cheaper to buy berries frozen, the fiber content is often nearly identical, making frozen berries a good smoothie ingredient. Avoid all fruit juices that don't contain pulp as this is where the vast majority of fiber resides.

Food	Fiber per medium fruit or cup if stated	Fiber per 100 grams	Cost
Avocado	13.5	6.7	$$$
Raspberries	8 per cup	6.5	$$
Blackberries	7.6 per cup	5.3	$
Dried Cranberries	4 per cup	5.3	$$
Pomegranate	11.3	4	$$
Pears	5.5	3.1	$
Dried Fig	1.5	2.9	$$
Bananas	3.1	2.6	$
Oranges	3.1	2.4	$
Blueberries	3.6 per cup	2.4	$
Red Delicious Apples	4.9	2.3	$
Strawberries	3.3 per cup	2	$

Vegetables

As a general rule, darker vegetables contain more fiber. As with fruit, do not remove the skin to optimize fiber intake. Vegetables mostly comprised of water, such as iceberg lettuce, and overcooked vegetables contain low amounts of fiber.

Food	Fiber per cup	Fiber per 100 grams	Cost
Artichoke	7.7	5.4	$$
Parsnips	6.5	4.9	$
Collards	1.4	4	$
Brussel Sprouts	4.1	3.8	$
Kale	2.6	3.6	$
Broccoli	5.1	3.3	$
Sweet Potatoes	6.6	3.3	$
Butternut squash	6.6	3.2	$
Carrots	4.7	3	$
Eggplant	2.5	3	$
Asparagus	2.8	2.1	$$
Beets	3.4	2	$
Leeks	1.6	1.8	$

Legumes

Legumes price vary dramatically depending on whether they're bought dried or canned. If dried, they often require a lot of preparation before cooking. Some dried beans require 10 hours of soaking plus an additional few hours of simmering before being edible. Dried beans can be bought in larger quantities since they often grow tremendously in size after being exposed to water: dried chickpeas tripling in size after being soaked and boiled. Since dried beans and canned beans vary in price dramatically, there is not a cost category for this section. Please note, most recipes in this book state that the legumes come from a can, as they are precooked and are much easier to work with.

Food	Fiber per cup	Fiber per 100 grams
White Beans	18.6	10.4
Kidney Beans	16.5	9.3
Pinto Beans	15.4	9
Black Beans	15	8.7
Split Peas	16.3	8.3
Lentils	15.6	7.9
Chickpeas	12.5	7.6
Black-eyed Peas	11.1	6.5
Peas	8.3	5.7
Baked Beans	13.9	5.5
Lima Beans	9.2	5.4
Refried Beans	11.4	4.7

Nuts and Seeds

Nuts and seeds are overwhelmingly fibrous and packed with nutrients. They are also high in calories and Omega 6, which can cause inflammation if not balanced with Omega 3. As with everything, moderation is key.

Food	Fiber per cup	Fiber per 100 grams	Cost
Chia Seeds	9.8	34.4	$$
Flax Seeds	7.8	27.3	$$$
Almonds	3.6	12.5	$$

Food	Fiber per cup	Fiber per 100 grams	Cost
Sunflower Seeds	3.2	11.1	$
Pistachios	3	10.6	$$$
Hazelnuts	2.8	9.7	$$$
Pecans	2.7	9.6	$$$
Dry Roasted Peanuts	2.4	9.4	$
Brazil Nuts	2.1	7.5	$$$
Walnuts	5.4	6.7	$$$

Intestinal Flora Diversification

Probiotics

It's difficult to produce probiotic rich food as bacteria need to live in specific states to survive and grow. Fermentation is the process of allowing bacteria or yeast to breakdown carbohydrates over a period of time, feeding the bacteria and allowing it to multiply. Even if a product is fermented, applying moderate amounts of heat to the product can kill off healthy bacteria.

Probiotic-rich Foods

Food	Description	Cost
Kefir	Kefir is a fermented probiotic drink that's produced by adding cultures of bacteria and yeast to goat or cow's milk. It's one of the best sources of probiotics.	$
Greek or Probiotic Yogurt	Check food labelling to ensure the yogurt contains live or active cultures. Bacteria is easily killed off and the manufacturer will have to produce the yogurt with as little	$

Food	Description	Cost
	heat as possible. Try to avoid artificially sweetened yogurts.	
Miso Soup or Paste	A Japanese seasoning made from fermenting soybeans with salt and a type of fungus.	$
Tempeh	Another fermented soybean that consists of a nutty, firm patty. The fermentation process adds vitamin B12 which soybeans do not naturally contain as B12 is found in meat, fish and dairy. Tempeh is a smart choice for vegetarians.	$$
Traditional Buttermilk	Buttermilk can be misleading. There are two types, traditional and cultured. Traditional buttermilk is the leftover liquid from making butter and is consumed in India, Nepal & Pakistan. This type of buttermilk contains a thorough source of probiotics. Cultured buttermilk is fermented pasteurized low-fat or non-fat milk. The pasteurization process kills off healthy bacteria. Cultured buttermilk found in American supermarkets do not contain probiotics.	$$$
Sauerkraut	Sauerkraut is fermented cabbage. The taste can vary dramatically depending on the producer but is defined by its sour & salty taste. Only buy unpasteurized sauerkraut as pasteurization kills live bacteria.	$

Food	Description	Cost
Kimchi	Kimchi is a mixture of fermented cabbage, chili flakes and other vegetables such as garlic and scallion. It's normally eaten as a side dish in Korea or fried together with rice.	$$
Kombucha	Kombucha is a fermented black or green tea drink. However, high heat is known to kill bacteria and there's a lack of high-quality evidence proving the probiotic benefits of kombucha.	$$
Pickles	Pickles that are created from pickled cucumber in salt and water contain healthy probiotics. Cucumbers pickled in vinegar do not contain probiotics.	$
Gouda, Mozzarella, Cheddar & Cottage Cheese	It's important to look for live or active cultures on food labels before buying cheese. Not all cheese contains probiotics.	$$
Red Wine	Alcohol is highly toxic and any form of excess alcohol damages the gut. However, due to the high number of polyphenols contained in red wine, it's been observed that low to moderate consumption increased healthy bacteria and decreased harmful bacteria. Avoiding alcohol altogether is the best option, but if you must choose, red wine is the only type of alcohol with this positive effect.	$$

Probiotic-harming Foods

Food	Description
Alcohol	All excessive forms of alcohol are harmful to the gut microbiome.
Artificial Sweeteners	Artificial sweetener fed mice have been observed with reduced levels of good gut bacteria. Research is in its initial stages and the same results haven't been consistently observed in humans. It appears that consuming artificial sweeteners over sugar has some negative effects in some people, and no effects in others. More research is needed.

Prebiotics

Prebiotics refer to the dietary fiber that feeds healthy bacteria, helping them to survive and grow. Some types of Dietary Fibers include Inulin, Fructooligosaccharides (FOS), Beta-glucan, Arabinoxylan Oligosaccharides (AXOS) and Galacto-oligosaccharides (GOS)[55]. Fibrous vegetables are a major source of prebiotics alongside select fruits. Foods without dietary fiber, such as processed snacks, meat or dairy, contain limited or zero prebiotic benefits.

Food	Prebiotic Fiber	Cost
Sunchokes aka Jerusalem Artichokes	Inulin and FOS	$$
Garlic	Inulin and FOS	$
Onions	Inulin and FOS	$
Leeks	Inulin and FOS	$
Asparagus	Inulin and FOS	$$
Bananas	Inulin and FOS	$
Sweet Potatoes	Inulin and FOS	$$$

Food	Prebiotic Fiber	Cost
Oats	Beta-glucan	$
Apples	Pectin, Sorbitol & Mannitol	$
Flaxseed	Mucilage & Lignin	$$$
Beans and Peas	GOS	$

Vitamin C

Vitamin C is a powerful antioxidant, having a positive impact on skin health, immune function and gastrointestinal health, to name a few. Vitamin C is not produced by the body and cannot be stored, which means it's important to regularly consume a sufficient quantity every day. The recommended daily value (DV) is 75-90mg. Aside from the well-known abundance of vitamin C contained in citrus fruits, some lesser known alternatives are peppers, some herbs and vegetables.

Food	% of Vitamin C DV per Cup	% of Vitamin C DV per 100g	Cost
Green Chili Peppers	404%	269%	$
Guava	419%	254%	$$$
Bell Peppers	303%	204%	$
Thyme	1 Tsp = 1%	178%	$
Parsley	1 Tsp = 1%	148%	$
Jalapeno Peppers	119%	132%	$
Kale	17%	104%	$$
Kiwifruit	185%	103%	$
Broccoli	90%	99%	$
Canned Pimentos	181%	94%	$
Brussel Sprouts	83%	94%	$

Food	% of Vitamin C DV per Cup	% of Vitamin C DV per 100g	Cost
Grapefruit	38%	88%	$$
Cayenne Pepper	1 Tsp = 1%	85%	$
Papaya	98%	68%	$$
Strawberries	99%	65%	$$
Oranges	180%	59%	$
Lemons	125%	59%	$
Garden Peas	64%	44%	$
Sugar Apples	48%	40%	$
Cooked Tomatoes	61%	25%	$

Help Shape Our Books

If this book has helped you at all, I'd love to read your feedback on Amazon. Reviews help us refine our books, making our next one that little bit more helpful.

If you'd like to stay up-to-date with our publications, or would just like to drop us a message, feel free to email us at info.healthful@gmail.com. You can also follow us on www.facebook.com/healthfulpublications. Thanks for reading so far and we hope you enjoy the recipes!

Recipes

This section takes the most beneficial ingredients from the previous section and suggests recipes for breakfast, lunch and dinner. Their exact benefits are broken down, alongside their macronutrients and estimated value. The macronutrients are taken from U.S. Department of Agriculture, Agricultural Research Service, FoodData Central, fdc.nal.usda.gov. All recipes contain both US Imperial and Metric measurements for readers all around the world.

Please note, the value calculation is a rough estimation as prices for ingredients vary depending on season, location and producer. There is also a difference between the total cost of a meal's ingredients and the price per macronutrients. For example, Flax seeds can be quite expensive, but they provide fiber, prebiotics and Omega 3. Therefore, the money spent on flax seeds provides 3x the benefit as the money spent on another ingredient.

Breakfast

Crunchy Fruit Pot

Macronutrients & Omegas per Serving

Kcal:	423	Carbs:		51.5g	Vitamin C	77mg
Fat:	15.2g	Fiber:		12.3g	% of DV	86%
Protein:	23.5g	Cholesterol:		20mg		

Boasting a high amount of fiber and prebiotics from the oats and fruit, as well as a source of probiotics from the yogurt. If adding additional fruit, make sure to leave the skin intact to keep as much of the fiber and prebiotics as possible. Flax seeds can be switched to chia seeds for a cheaper alternative.

Benefits: Fiber, Prebiotics, Probiotics & Vitamin C

Value: $$

Time: 5 mins

Serves: 1

Ingredients

1 Kiwifruit
1/3 Cup (50g) Raspberries
1/4 Cup (40g) Oats
3/4 Cup (150g) Greek Yogurt
1 Tbsp Flax seed

Method

1. Mix the flax seeds, oats and Greek yogurt in a bowl.

2. Slice the kiwifruit and add it to the bottom of a separate bowl or wide glass. Top the kiwifruit with the yogurt mixture. Add the berries on top and serve.

Apple & Grapefruit Porridge

Macronutrients & Omegas per Serving

Kcal:	391	Carbs:	70.6g	Vitamin C	34mg
Fat:	7.5g	Fiber:	10.3g	**% of DV**	38%
Protein:	12g	Cholesterol:	13mg		

A warm wintery breakfast that'll leave you satiated for the whole morning. Both the oats and apple contain fiber and prebiotics to feed your good gut bacteria and allow for easy digestion.

Benefits: Fiber, Prebiotics & Vitamin C

Value: $

Time: Less than 10 mins

Serves: 4

Ingredients

3 Grapefruits

4 Red Delicious Apples

1 Cup (160g) Oats

2 1/4 Cups (500ml) Whole Milk

1 Tsp Ground Cinnamon

Method

1. Core and dice the apples. Cut each grapefruit in two halves. Put 3 halves aside. With the other 3 halves, use a knife to trace along the membranes of each segment of grapefruit to loosen them.

2. Add the oats and milk to a small saucepan, bring to boil then simmer. Squeeze 3 halves of the grapefruit that were left to one side into the saucepan, stir and simmer for 2 more mins, stirring occasionally.

3. Spoon in the loose grapefruit membranes, apples and cinnamon, cooking for an additional 2 mins until the porridge is creamy. You can save some grapefruit sections for topping if desired. Serve hot.

Whole Wheat Banana Bread

Macronutrients & Omegas per Serving

Kcal:	573	Carbs:	93.3g	Vitamin C	8mg
Fat:	21.2g	Fiber:	8.1g	% of DV	9%
Protein:	10.8g	Cholesterol:	82mg		

A fantastic way to use up any overripe bananas. This delicious bread is full of fiber and prebiotics from the whole wheat flour and bananas.

Benefits: Fiber & Prebiotics

Value: $

Time: 1 Hour 45 mins

Serves: 4

Ingredients

2 Eggs

3 Mashed Banana (354g)

1/4 Cup (60ml) Hot Water

1/2 Cup (170g) Honey

1 3/4 Cups (210g) Whole Wheat Flour

1/2 Tsp Salt

1/2 Tsp Cinnamon, Plus More for Topping

1 Tsp Vanilla Extract

1 Tsp Baking Soda

5 Tbsp Olive Oil

Method

1. Preheat oven to 325°F (165°C)/gas 3 and grease a 9×5-inch (23x13cm) loaf pan.

2. Add oil, honey, 1/4 cup water & 1 tsp baking soda into a large bowl and mix well. After mixing, add the eggs and beat thoroughly.

3. Add the mashed bananas, vanilla, salt and cinnamon into the bowl, stir well. Finally stir in the flour until combined.

4. Pour the batter evenly into the greased loaf pan.

5. Sprinkle with cinnamon, you can use a toothpick or the tip of a butter knife to make a pattern.

6. Bake for 60 mins. Check the bread is done by inserting a toothpick in the top, if it doesn't come out dry, bake for an additional 5 mins. Remove from oven and leave it to cool for 5 mins in the pan. Transfer it to a wire rack to cool for 30 minutes before serving.

Note: Recipe adapted from cookieandkate.com

Blackberry, Apple & Orange Oat Bake

Macronutrients & Omegas per Serving

Kcal:	412	Carbs:		50.1g	Vitamin C	35mg
Fat:	19.2g	Fiber:		11g	% of DV	39%
Protein:	13.8g	Cholesterol:		38mg		

A delicious, fruity baked breakfast that can be made ahead of time in batches. Maple syrup will give this breakfast dish a more dessert-like feel. Be sure to use fresh milk as older milk is acidic, and milk curdles if it's heated in an acidic environment.

Benefits: Fiber, Prebiotics, Probiotics & Vitamin C

Value: $$

Time: 1 Hour

Serves: 6

Ingredients

1 Egg
2 Red Delicious Apples
2 Oranges
6 Cardamom Pods, Bashed or 1/4 Tsp Ground Cardamom
1 Cup (100g) Pecans
1 1/4 Cup (200g) Oats
2 1/4 Cups (320g) Blackberries
17floz (500ml) Fresh Whole Milk
1 Tsp (4g) Ground Cinnamon
1 Tsp Vanilla Extract
1 Tsp Baking Powder
Greek Yogurt to Serve

Method

1. Heat the oven to 400°F (200°C)/350°F (180°C) fan/ gas 6. Core and cut the apples into 0.5-inch (1cm) cubes; chop the pecans; beat the egg; remove the skin and pith from the oranges, cutting the oranges into roughly 1/4-inch (0.5cm) rounds.

2. Add the apple, spices and milk into a small saucepan. Cover and gently bring to a boil, simmering for 10 mins. Take off the heat and allow it to infuse for 15 mins minimum.

3. Discard the spice. Pour the mixture into a large bowl and crush the apples with the back of a fork. Mix in the beaten egg, oats, vanilla, baking powder, pecans and blackberries.

4. Place half of the orange rounds on the bottom of a 2-quart (2-liter) ovenproof dish and then evenly pour in the mixture, bake for 15 mins. Place the remaining orange rounds on top and back for a further 15 mins or until the middle is piping hot. Serve with yogurt.

Breakfast Burrito

Macronutrients & Omegas per Serving

Kcal:	418	Carbs:	40.7g	Vitamin C	90mg
Fat:	22.1g	Fiber:	13g	% of DV	100%
Protein:	14.4g	Cholesterol:	166mg		

Full of healthy fats from the avocado and a little spicy tang from the chipotle paste. This is a perfect dish to make two days in a row to finish off the avocado...although the taste may have you making a second helping immediately.

Benefits: Fiber, Probiotics & Vitamin C

Value: $$

Time: 5 mins

Serves: 1

Ingredients

½ Small Avocado, Stoned & Peeled

1 Egg

1 Whole Wheat Tortilla Wrap

7 Cherry Tomatoes (200g)

3 Cups (50g) Kale

1 Tsp (5g) Chipotle Paste

1 Tsp Olive Oil

1 Tbsp Greek Yogurt

Method

1. Halve the cherry tomatoes and slice the avocado. Add the egg, a little salt and pepper as well as the chipotle paste to a bowl. Whisk until the egg is airy.

2. Heat the oil on a medium heat in a large frying pan.

3. Add the kale and tomatoes, cooking until the tomatoes have softened and the kale has reduced in size. Move them to one side of the pan.

4. Pour the egg and chipotle mixture into the empty half of the pan and scramble.

5. Warm the wrap then spoon in Greek yogurt, eggs, kale and tomatoes evenly to the center. Finally, top with avocado and serve.

Smoked Salmon & Tomato Omelet

Macronutrients & Omegas per Serving

Kcal:	298	Carbs:		12.5g	Vitamin C	22mg
Fat:	16g	Fiber:		2.4g	% of DV	24%
Protein:	25.7g	Cholesterol:		354mg		

A high protein meal that's healthy for the brain and gut bacteria. Omelets are versatile, allowing you to add or remove vegetables or meat depending on your goal.

Benefits: Prebiotics & Probiotics
Value: $$$
Time: 10 mins
Serves: 2

Ingredients

Butter to Grease the Pan
1/4 Cup (25g) Shredded Cheddar Cheese
1 Onion (110g)
2 Tomatoes (246g)
4 Eggs
3.5oz (100g) Smoked Salmon
1 Tsp Chopped Parsley
1 Tsp Chopped Basil
2 Tbsp (60ml) Whole Milk

Method

1. Add the butter to a non-stick frying pan and warm on medium heat, tilting the pan until the melted butter covers the entire bottom.

2. Beat the eggs and herbs together in a bowl, add a pinch of salt and pepper. Finely dice the onion.

3. Cook the onions for 3 mins and then add the tomatoes, cooking for another 2 mins until they start to soften. Add the eggs and herb mixture.

4. Stir the eggs gently allowing uncooked egg on the surface of the mixture to fall to the base of the pan between cooked egg. Once there's no visible raw egg, stop stirring and allow the mixture to cook into an omelet.

5. Add the smoked salmon to the center of the omelet and sprinkle with cheese. Cook for 30 seconds. Continue cooking the omelet to your desired texture.

6. Once finished, slowly tilt the pan and move one side of the omelet to a plate, folding over the farthest side so the salmon is neatly tucked in the middle. Serve immediately.

Apple & Cardamom Quinoa Porridge

Macronutrients & Omegas per Serving

Kcal:	400	Carbs:	70.7g	Vitamin C	0mg
Fat:	7.8g	Fiber:	8.9g	% of DV	0%
Protein:	12.1g	Cholesterol:	13mg		

A flavorful twist on the classic porridge. The red delicious apples can be switched out for different ripe fruit, just make sure they contain plenty of prebiotics. Remove the maple syrup if you prefer a savory breakfast.

Benefits: Fiber & Prebiotics

Value: $$

Time: 20 mins

Serves: 2

Ingredients

2 Red Delicious Apples

4 Cardamom Pods

1oz (25g) Oats

2.5oz (75g) Quinoa

8.5floz (250ml) Fresh Whole Milk

1 Tsp Maple Syrup

Method

1. Add 3.5floz (100ml) of milk and 8.5floz (250ml) of water into a small saucepan. Add the cardamom pods, quinoa and oats. Bring to a boil then simmer gently for 15 mins, stirring occasionally to stop the bottom of the pan from burning the quinoa or oats.

2. Pour in the remaining milk and cook for an additional 5 mins until creamy. While cooking, cut the apples into slices.

3. Remove the cardamom pods, pour into bowls and top with the apples and maple syrup.

Overnight Apple & Banana Muesli

Macronutrients & Omegas per Serving

Kcal:	399	Carbs:	61g	Vitamin C	6mg
Fat:	13.5g	Fiber:	9.6g	% of DV	7%
Protein:	13.3g	Cholesterol:	7mg		

A breakfast that requires no cooking and can be made the night before ahead of a busy day. Filled to the brim with plenty of fiber, prebiotics and probiotics.

Benefits: Fiber,
   Prebiotics &
   Probiotics
Value: $$$
Time: 5 mins
Serves: 2

Ingredients
1 Red Delicious Apple
1 Banana
1 Walnut
1 Brazil Nut
4 Hazelnuts
1/3 Cup (50g) Oats
1/2 Tsp Ground
   Cinnamon
2 Tsp Sunflower
   Seeds
2 Tsp Pumpkin Seeds
1 Tbsp Flax Seeds
3 Tbsp Sultanas
5 1/2 Tbsp Greek
   Yogurt

Method

1. Chop the brazil nuts, hazelnuts and walnuts. Slice the banana.

2. Grate the red delicious apple into a bowl and add the cinnamon, oats, seeds and half the nuts. Stir together well.

3. Add the yogurt and 3.5floz (100ml) cold water, stir well and then cover and chill the mixture overnight or for a few hours.

4. When ready to eat, spoon the muesli into 2 bowls, top with the sultanas, banana and remaining nuts.

Strawberry & Avocado Smoothie

Macronutrients & Omegas per Serving

Kcal:	207	Carbs:	17.8g	Vitamin C	49mg
Fat:	12.7g	Fiber:	4.9g	% of DV	54%
Protein:	7.9g	Cholesterol:	15mg		

A sharp and fruity pick-me-up that can be drank on the commute to work or as an afternoon snack. Smoothies are far cheaper to make yourself than to order at a smoothie stand, it also allows you to switch out sugar-filled yogurt for probiotic-filled Greek yogurt.

Benefits: Probiotics & Vitamin C

Value: $$$

Time: 5 mins

Serves: 4

Method

1. Simply add all the ingredients into a blender and blend until smooth. Add a little water if too thick and blend again.

Ingredients

Squeeze of Lemon or Lime Juice

1 Avocado, Stoned, Peeled & Cut into Chunks

1/2 Cup (140g) Greek Yogurt

2 Cups (300g) Strawberries

13.5floz (400ml) Whole Milk

1 Tsp (7g) Honey

Nutty Bread with Seeds and Dried Fig served with Cottage Cheese and Apple

Macronutrients & Omegas per Serving

Kcal:	400	Carbs:	53.1g	Vitamin C	1mg
Fat:	17.8g	Fiber:	8.3g	% of DV	1%
Protein:	13.7g	Cholesterol:	34mg		

This crispy, nutty bread is a supercharged version of whole wheat bread. Containing the regular high dose of fiber that you get with whole wheat bread but pushed to its prebiotic and probiotic limit. This loaf will last in the fridge for 1 month.

Benefits: Fiber, Prebiotics & Probiotics

Value: $$$

Time: 1 Hour 30

Serves: 8

Ingredients

1 Large Egg

1 Red Delicious Apple

12 Dried Figs (100g), Thinly Sliced

1/3 Cup (50g) Oats

3/4 Cup (75g) Walnuts

1 1/2 Cups (200g) Self-Raising Whole Wheat Flour

1oz (30g each) Almonds, Brazil Nuts & Hazelnuts

1oz (25g) Cottage Cheese Per Person

5oz (140g) Sultanas

13.5floz (400ml) Hot Black Tea

1 Tsp Baking Powder

1 Tbsp + 2 Tsp (16g) Flax Seeds

3 Tbsp (25g) Pumpkin Seed

Method

1. Heat oven to 350°F (170°C)/300°F (150°C) fan/gas mark 3 1/2.

2. Add the oats, sultanas and figs into a large bowl with the hot tea, stir well and put to one side.

3. Line the base and sides of a 2lb (1kg) loaf tin with baking parchment. Separate 1/2 Cup (50g) of walnuts and the 2 tsp of flax seeds from the rest of the nuts and seeds, these will be used in the topping later. In a bowl add the flour, baking powder and the remaining nuts and seeds that won't be used for topping. Stir well.

4. Beat the egg into the cooled fruity tea mixture, add the flour and seeds mixture and stir well. Pour into the tin, make sure the top is level. Place the rest of the walnuts and flax seeds on top.

5. Bake for 1 hour then cover the top with foil and bake for 15 mins longer. A toothpick inserted into the center of the loaf should come out clean.

6. Remove from the tin, leaving the parchment on until the loaf has cooled, and the parchment is cold.

7. When ready to serve, cut into slices, spread with cottage cheese and slices of apple.

Lunch

Lentil & Sweet Potato Soup

Macronutrients & Omegas per Serving

Kcal:	339	Carbs:	56.4g	Vitamin C	31mg
Fat:	9.4g	Fiber:	8.7g	% of DV	34%
Protein:	9g	Cholesterol:	5mg		

A hearty and slightly spicy soup packed with prebiotics from sweet potatoes and lentils. Soups are great for cooking in batches.

Benefits: Fiber, Prebiotics & Vitamin C

Value: $$

Time: 35 mins

Serves: 6

Ingredients

Thumb-Size (16g) Fresh Ginger

1 Lime

1 Green Chili Pepper Sweet or Spicy (48g)

1 Red Delicious Apple (210g)

2 Onions (220g)

3 Garlic Cloves

7 Sweet Potatoes (900g)

1/2 cup (100g) Red Lentils

1 1/4 Cup (20g) Cilantro

10floz (300ml) Whole Milk

1.25qt (1.2L) Vegetable Stock

2 Tsp Medium Curry Powder

3 Tbsp Olive Oil

Method

1. Roughly chop the onions, red apples, ginger and pepper, crush the garlic and chop the cilantro stalks. Finely dice the sweet potatoes.

2. Toast the curry powder in a large saucepan over a medium heat for 2 mins. Add the olive oil, gently stirring as it sizzles. Add the garlic, onions, apple, cilantro stalks and a pinch of salt and pepper. Cook gently for 5 mins, stirring occasionally.

3. Add the sweet potatoes to the pan alongside the stock, milk, lentils and pepper. Cover and simmer for 20 mins.

4. Blend until creamy. Juice the lime into the soup, check the seasoning and serve. Top with chopped cilantro leaves.

Tomato Soup with Pasta

Macronutrients & Omegas per Serving

Kcal:	453	Carbs:	68.1g	Vitamin C	13mg
Fat:	14.5g	Fiber:	12.7g	% of DV	14%
Protein:	17.1g	Cholesterol:	0mg		

A vegetable packed tomato soup that'll fill you with nutrients as well as prebiotics. The chickpeas, pasta and bread will keep you full until dinner.

Benefits: Fiber & Prebiotics

Value: $

Time: 30 mins

Serves: 4

Ingredients

1 Onion (110g)
2 Celery Sticks (80g)
2 Garlic Cloves
4 Slices (128g) Whole Wheat Bread
2/3 Cup (150g) Whole Wheat Pasta
14oz (400g) Can Chopped Tomatoes
14oz (400g) Can Chickpeas
24floz (700ml) Vegetable Stock
1 Tbsp Tomato Purée
2 Tbsp Basil Pesto
2 Tbsp Olive Oil

Method

1. Heat the olive oil in a large saucepan and chop the onion and celery. Crush the garlic. Fry the onion and celery for 8 mins then add the garlic and cook for 1 more min. Put the pesto and oil aside and stir in all of the other ingredients.

2. Bring to a boil and then reduce the heat and leave to simmer for 7 mins or until the pasta is tender. Season.

3. Mix the pesto with the last tablespoon of oil. Pour the soup into bowls and drizzle the pesto mixture over the soup. Serve with bread.

Lentil Soup

Macronutrients & Omegas per Serving

Kcal:	317	Carbs:	60.6g	**Vitamin C**	44mg
Fat:	2.4g	**Fiber:**	10g	**% of DV**	49%
Protein:	15.1g	**Cholesterol:**	0mg		

Another lunch-suitable soup that's extremely easy to prepare and will boil for an hour in peace. Leeks and red lentils are the prebiotic powerhouses of this dish, ready to feed your good gut bacteria.

Benefits: Fiber and Prebiotics

Value: $

Time: 1 Hour 10

Serves: 4

Ingredients

1 Green Chili Pepper Sweet or Spicy (45g)

2 Large Leeks (270g)

4 Slices (128g) Whole Wheat Bread

6 Carrots (366g)

3/4 Cup (150g) Red Lentils

2qt (2L) Vegetable Stock

2 Tbsp (8g) Parsley

Method

1. Finely chop the carrots, pepper and parsley. Slice the leeks.

2. Add the stock and lentils to a large saucepan and bring to a boil for a few mins.

3. Add the leeks, carrots and pepper and season to taste. Bring to a simmer and cover it for 45-60 mins until the lentils are broken down.

4. Scatter with parsley and serve with a slice of buttered whole wheat bread.

Miso Soup

Macronutrients & Omegas per Serving

Kcal:	184	Carbs:	19.1g	Vitamin C	11mg
Fat:	6g	Fiber:	4g	% of DV	12%
Protein:	18.7g	Cholesterol:	0mg		

Miso soup is a cheap and quick way to fill your stomach with more healthy probiotics. This soup is the definition of umami.

Benefits: Probiotics

Value: $

Time: 15 mins

Serves: 2

Ingredients

1 Sheet (28g) Dried
  Seaweed
1/4 Cup (62g) Firm
  Tofu
1/2 Cup (32g) Swiss
  Chard
1/2 Cup (45g) Scallion
1qt (950ml)
  Vegetable Stock
4 Tbsp Miso Paste

Method

1. Chop the swiss chard and scallion. Dice the tofu into cubes.

2. Simmer the vegetable stock in a medium saucepan. Add the dried seaweed and simmer for 5 mins.

3. Place miso into a small bowl and add a little hot water. Whisk until smooth then set aside.

4. Add the swiss chard, scallion and tofu into the saucepan for 5 mins. Once cooked, remove from the heat and add the resting miso paste. Serve and eat immediately.

Lima Bean & Leek Soup topped with Kale, Toasted Hazelnuts & Bacon

Macronutrients & Omegas per Serving

Kcal:	334	Carbs:	34.8g	Vitamin C	36mg
Fat:	18.2g	Fiber:	7.2g	% of DV	40%
Protein:	10.2g	Cholesterol:	14mg		

An elaborate soup for those that want a mixture of textures in every bite. It contains a healthy fusion of vegetables, beans, nuts, meat and leafy greens full of prebiotics.

Benefits: Prebiotics & Vitamin C

Value: $$$

Time: 40 mins

Serves: 4

Ingredients

3 Rashers (84g) Streaky Bacon

5 Leeks (500g)

1/4 Cup (28g) Hazelnuts

2 1/2 Cups (40g) Chopped Kale

2 X 14oz (400g) Can Lima Beans

16floz (500ml) Vegetable Stock

2 Tsp Chopped Thyme

2 Tsp Mustard

1 Tbsp Chopped Parsley

1 Tbsp + 1 Tsp Olive Oil

Method

1. Slice the leeks, chop the hazelnuts and kale whilst removing any tough kale stems.

2. Add 1 tbsp oil into a large saucepan and heat over a low heat. Add the thyme, leeks and seasoning. Cover and cook for 15 mins, the leeks should be soft. If the leeks stick together in the pan, add a splash of water. Add both cans of lima beans, water included, the stock and mustard. Bring to a boil and simmer for 3 mins. Take off the heat and blend to make a soup. Add the parsley, adjust the seasoning if necessary and give it a stir. Keep to one side.

3. Add the bacon to a large, non-stick frying pan and cook until crispy over a medium heat for 3-4 mins. Set the bacon aside to cool but keep the bacon grease in the pan and add the last tsp oil. Add the kale and hazelnuts and cook for 2 mins, stirring until the kale is wilted and crisping at the edges and the hazelnuts are toasted. Cut the cooled bacon into small pieces and add into the kale mixture, stirring thoroughly.

4. When ready to serve, reheat the soup and add some water if too thick. Serve in bowls, placing the kale, hazelnut and bacon mixture on top.

Quinoa Tabbouleh

Macronutrients & Omegas per Serving

Kcal:	326	Carbs:	48.7g	Vitamin C	88mg
Fat:	11g	Fiber:	8g	% of DV	98%
Protein:	11.1g	Cholesterol:	0mg		

A fresh and tangy quinoa-based lunch. Although light, it's sure to refresh and keep you alert for the rest of the afternoon.

Benefits: Fiber, Prebiotics & Vitamin C

Value: $$

Time: 40 mins

Serves: 2

Ingredients

1/3 Cucumber (100g)
1/2 Garlic Clove
Juice and Zest 1/2 Lemon
3 Tomatoes (300g)
Drop of Vanilla Extract
Pinch of Himalayan Pink Salt
1/2 Cup (100g) Quinoa
1 1/4 Cup (75g) Chopped Parsley
2 1/2 Cups (50g) Arugula Leaves
1 Tbsp Olive Oil
2 Tbsp Balsamic Vinegar

Method

1. Cut the tomatoes and cucumber into smaller than bite-sized cubes, around 0.5-inch (1cm) and crush the garlic.

2. Cook the quinoa as per its instructions & set aside to cool. Once cooked move onto step 3, if no instructions are present follow the rest of this step. Rinse the quinoa in a fine mesh colander under 30 seconds and drain well to remove the bitterness. Add the quinoa to a saucepan alongside 1 cup water, keep uncovered. Bring to a boil and then simmer for 10 mins or until all the water has been absorbed. Remove from the heat and cover, allowing to steam for 5 mins.

3. Whisk the vinegar, olive oil, lemon juice, vanilla, salt and garlic in a jug until smooth.

4. Mix together with the quinoa and serve on top of the arugula.

Spring Tabbouleh

Macronutrients & Omegas per Serving

Kcal:	593	Carbs:	75.4g	Vitamin C	58mg
Fat:	26.8g	Fiber:	17.3g	% of DV	64%
Protein:	19.3g	Cholesterol:	0mg		

A different take on the tabbouleh, raising the fiber content with the addition of both oats and buckwheat. This version includes oven-baking so is perfect for kitchen cleaning multi-tasking. The herbs and lemon add that sharp tabbouleh tang.

Benefits: Fiber, Prebiotics & Vitamin C

Value: $$

Time: 45 mins

Serves: 4

Ingredients

1 Cucumber (300g)
2 Lemons, Zested and Juiced
14 Large (250g) Radishes
3/4 Cup (125g) Oats
3/4 Cup (125g) Buckwheat
1 1/2 Cups (240g) Frozen Peas
1/4 Cup (43g) Pomegranate Seeds, To Serve
14oz (400g) Canned Chickpeas
1 Tbsp Garam Masala
4 Tbsp Parsley
4 Tbsp Mint
6 Tbsp Olive Oil

Method

1. Zest and juice the lemons. Chop the radishes, cucumbers, parsley and mint.

2. Preheat the oven to 400°F (200°C)/360°F (180°C) fan/gas 6. Put the chickpeas in a large roast tin, add 4 tbsp oil, garam masala and some seasoning. Thoroughly mix until the chickpeas are coated. Cook for 15 mins, the chickpeas should be starting to crisp. Add the peas, lemon zest, oats and buckwheat, mix thoroughly. Bake for another 10 mins.

3. Transfer to a large mixing bowl and add the herbs, radishes, cucumber, oil and lemon juice. Mix thoroughly. Serve with pomegranate seeds.

Kale, Bulgur & Hazelnut Tabbouleh

Macronutrients & Omegas per Serving

Kcal:	512	Carbs:	76.4g	Vitamin C	63mg
Fat:	15.2g	Fiber:	14.9g	% of DV	70%
Protein:	24.8g	Cholesterol:	172mg		

The end of our lunchtime tabbouleh section and this time with bulgur, bringing it back to its classic taste. The yogurt is added, not only to balance out the dry texture of the bulgur, but to add some probiotics as well.

Benefits: Fiber, Prebiotics, Probiotics & Vitamin C

Value: $$

Time: 30 mins

Serves: 2

Ingredients

1/4 Garlic Clove
Juice and Zest 1 Lemon
1 Carrot (60g)
2 Eggs (88g)
3 Scallion (45g)
1/3 Cup (50g) Pomegranate Seeds
3/4 Cup (150g) Bulgur Wheat
3 3/4 Cups (60g) Kale
1 Tsp Chili Flakes
1 Tbsp Chopped Dill
1 Tbsp Chopped Mint
2 Tbsp White Wine Vinegar
2 1/2 Tbsp (20g) Hazelnuts
7 Tbsp Greek Yogurt

Method

1. If the hazelnuts aren't bought roasted, lay them whole on a cookie sheet and roast at 350°F (175°C) degrees for 15 mins, watching closely as it doesn't take them long to go from brown to burnt. Wait until cooled then place them in a large clean kitchen towel and rub them until the skins fall off.

2. Chop the hazelnuts, kale, scallions, dill and mint. Julienne (cut into 1/8-inch thick strips) the carrot. Crush the garlic. Cook the bulgur as per its instructions.

3. Bring a pan of water to the boil and add the eggs. Cook for 6 mins, then place in cold water until cool. Peel and cut in half. Put the lemon juice, zest, Greek yogurt, white wine vinegar, dill, mint and garlic into a food processor or blender with 2 tbsp water and some salt. Blend until smooth.

4. Break up the bulgur with a fork and add the hazelnuts, kale, carrots, pomegranate seeds, chili and scallions. Toss with the dressing, then top with the eggs to serve.

Pasta Salad with Tuna

Macronutrients & Omegas per Serving

Kcal:	597	Carbs:	73.9g	Vitamin C	9mg
Fat:	21.6g	Fiber:	9.3g	% of DV	10%
Protein:	30.2g	Cholesterol:	43mg		

A quick and easy pasta dish that's a surefire way to balance out your healthy fats for the day.

Benefits: Fiber & Probiotics

Value: $

Time: 20 mins

Serves: 4

Ingredients

1 Celery (40g)

4.5oz (125g) Mozzarella Ball (125g)

15 Peppadew/Cherry/ Peppers (150g)

1/2 Cup (110g) Cherry Tomato

1 Cup (24g) Basil Leaves

3 Cups (350g) Orecchiette Pasta

5 Cups (100g) Arugula Leaves

6oz (170g) Tuna

1 Tbsp Caper

3 Tbsp Olive Oil

5 Tbsp Balsamic Vinegar

Method

1. Chop the peppers, halve the cherry tomatoes and slice the celery.

2. Cook the pasta as per its instructions. Drain and add to a large bowl alongside all other ingredients except the basil and mozzarella. Stir well and serve. Tear the mozzarella and top the pasta alongside the basil.

Pomegranate and Broad Bean Salad

Macronutrients & Omegas per Serving

Kcal:	504	Carbs:		61.1g	Vitamin C	22mg
Fat:	24.5g	Fiber:		23.7g	% of DV	24%
Protein:	19.8g	Cholesterol:		16mg		

A salad packed with herbs that's great for immediate consumption or travel...if you store the dressing separately! The pumpkin seeds, fennel and broad beans add some fiber and crunch to the salad.

Benefits: Fiber & Probiotics

Value: $$

Time: 25 mins

Serves: 6

Ingredients

Small Bunch Mint (10g)

4.5oz (125g) Mozzarella Ball

1 Fennel Bulb (230g)

1 Lemon

1 Cup (200g) Bulgur

1 Cup (20g) Arugula

1 1/4 Cups (200g) Pomegranate Seeds

1 1/2 Cups (350g) Broad Beans

1 Tbsp Dijon Mustard

2 Tbsp Chopped Parsley (10g)

2 Tbsp Chopped Dill (10g)

2 Tbsp (16g) Pumpkin Seeds

2 Tbsp Apple Cider Vinegar

5 Tbsp Extra Virgin Olive Oil

Method

1. Finely chop the mint, parsley and dill. Toast the bread. Quarter the fennel bulb, remove the core and thinly slice the quarters.

2. Boil enough water to just about cover the bulgur. Add the bulgur, boiling water and salt to a bowl and cover for 10 mins.

3. If this meal will be eaten at a later date, add the lemon zest, lemon juice, 5 tbs olive oil, 2 tbsp cider vinegar and 1 tbsp mustard to a small transportable container and shake vigorously. Otherwise, add these ingredients to a bowl and stir thoroughly.

4. Uncover the bulgur. If there's any water left, drain it. Add the fennel, herbs, pomegranate seeds, broad beans and pumpkin seeds and mix thoroughly. Pull the mozzarella into chunks and top alongside the arugula.

5. When ready to serve, drizzle the dressing and mix everything thoroughly.

Pesto Chicken Salad

Macronutrients & Omegas per Serving

Kcal:	378	Carbs:		16.2g	Vitamin C	82mg
Fat:	19.8g	Fiber:		6.9g	% of DV	91%
Protein:	36g	Cholesterol:		99mg		

The star of this dish is the homemade avocado pesto. It's delicious and will teach you how to make pesto that's both cheaper and fresher than store bought.

Benefits: Prebiotics & Vitamin C

Value: $$$

Time: 30 mins

Serves: 4

Ingredients

1 Red Onion (148g)

1 1/2 (250g) Broccoli

2 Raw Beets (165g)

3 Skinless Chicken Breasts (543g)

1 Cup (100g) Watercress

1 Tsp Flax Seeds

1 Tbsp + 2 Tsp Olive Oil

Avocado Pesto (or use store bought):

1/2 Garlic Clove

Juice and Zest 1/2 Lemon

1 Avocado (150g), Stoned & Peeled

1/4 Cup (25g) Walnuts

1 1/3 Cup (32g) Basil

Method

1. Grate the raw beets, crush the garlic, crumble the walnuts and thinly slice the red onion.

2. Boil the broccoli in a large saucepan for 2 mins. Drain then finish it off in a gridle or frying pan for 2-3 mins alongside 1/2 tsp olive oil. Set aside to cool.

3. Brush the chicken with 1 1/2 tsp of olive oil and either gridle or fry until cooked through, roughly 3-4 mins each side. Put to one side then slice once cooled.

4. For the avocado pesto, pick the leaves from the basil and add the rest into a food processor. Add the avocado, garlic, walnuts, 1 tbsp oil, 1 tbsp lemon juice, 2 tbsp cold water and some seasoning. Blend until it turns to a smooth paste.

5. Put the sliced red onion on a plate and pour over the rest of the lemon juice, leaving to stand for a few mins.

6. In a large mixing bowl, toss the watercress, broccoli, onion and lemon juice from the bottom of the plate.

7. Serve the salad mix from the mixing bowl. Top with beetroot, chicken, basil leaves, lemon zest and flax seeds. Put the pesto in a small bowl that can be shared.

Beetroot & Chickpea Pita

Macronutrients & Omegas per Serving

Kcal:	266	Carbs:	50.9g	Vitamin C	3mg
Fat:	3.3g	Fiber:	8.3g	% of DV	3%
Protein:	11.8g	Cholesterol:	2mg		

This quick pita recipe is preferably made and eaten immediately. However, if planning to store in a lunchbox and eat later in the day, make sure to store the filling separately from the pita to prevent it from getting soggy.

Benefits: Fiber, Prebiotics & Probiotics

Value: $

Time: 30 mins/10 min with pre-boiled beet

Serves: 2

Ingredients

1 Small Carrot (40g)

1 Beet (80g)

2 Large (130g) Whole Wheat Pita

4oz (120g) Canned Chickpeas

1 Tsp Harissa

2 Tbsp Greek Yogurt

Method

1. Boil the beet for 30-60 mins depending on the size. It should be tender enough for a fork to go through but not soft and mushy.

2. Grate the beet and carrot into a bowl. Add the chickpeas, harissa and 1 tbsp Greek yogurt. Mix together with the backside of a fork. Alternatively add this mixture to a blender and blend until a hummus like texture.

3. Cut an opening in the middle of the pitas and add the mixture. Garnish with 1 tbsp Greek yogurt.

Veggie Club Sandwich

Macronutrients & Omegas per Serving

Kcal:	485	Carbs:		60.8g	Vitamin C	52mg
Fat:	20.7g	Fiber:		12.2g	% of DV	58%
Protein:	17.7g	Cholesterol:		0mg		

Another – perfect for the lunchbox – treat if the wet hummus mixture is kept away from the bread until serving of course!

Benefits: Fiber & Vitamin C

Value: $

Time: 10 mins

Serves: 1

Ingredients

Small Squeeze Lemon Juice

1 Carrot (60g)

2 Tomatoes (246g)

3 Slices (96g) Whole Wheat Bread

1 Cup (35g) Watercress

1 Tbsp Olive Oil

2 Tbsp Hummus

Method

1. Grate the carrot and cut the tomatoes into thick slices. Toast the bread.

2. Mix the carrot, watercress, lemon juice and olive oil together in a small bowl.

3. After the bread is toasted, spread the hummus over each slice of toast.

4. Top 1 slice (hummus side up) with half the watercress mixture & tomatoes, then add the next slice and repeat one more time. Make sure the final slice is hummus side down, press down and slice into quarters.

Spicy Chicken Avocado Wraps

Macronutrients & Omegas per Serving

Kcal:	556	Carbs:		45.9g	Vitamin C	91mg
Fat:	25.7g	Fiber:		14.8g	% of DV	101%
Protein:	37.5g	Cholesterol:		77mg		

Leftover chicken in the fridge? Time to pair it with some avocado and bell pepper, wrapped in a whole wheat tortilla for a high protein and fiber lunch.

Benefits: Fiber, Prebiotics & Vitamin C

Value: $$$

Time: 15 mins

Serves: 2

Ingredients

1/2 Juice Lime
1 Chicken Breast (180g), Thinly Sliced at An Angle
1 Garlic Clove
1 Avocado (175g), Stoned & Peeled
1 Red Bell Pepper (120g)
2 Large Whole Wheat Wraps (140g)
1/2 Tsp Mild Chili Powder
1 Tsp Olive Oil
1 Tbsp Cilantro

Method

1. Chop the garlic and cilantro. Thinly slice the bell pepper and chicken.

2. Add the chicken breast to a bowl alongside the chili powder, garlic and lime juice. Stir thoroughly so the chicken is coated.

3. Add the oil to a non-stick frying pan and fry the chicken for a few mins until warmed through.

4. Warm the wraps on a gas stove top or in the microwave as per its instructions.

5. Add the peppers to the frying pan. Squash half an avocado into each wrap and then evenly split the contents of the frying pan into both wraps. Top with cilantro, roll the wraps and serve.

Crunchy Chickpea & Avocado Wraps

Macronutrients & Omegas per Serving

Kcal:	664	Carbs:	72.7g	Vitamin C	119mg
Fat:	34.5g	Fiber:	22.1g	% of DV	132%
Protein:	20.7g	Cholesterol:	5mg		

For the days where you can't seem to get your recommended fiber, fear not. This recipe catapults you into your 20-38g recommended fiber intake per day. If the combination of chickpeas and whole wheat tortillas is a little dry for your palette, liberally add more Greek yogurt or avocado.

Benefits: Fiber, Prebiotics, Probiotics & Vitamin C

Value: $$

Time: 45 mins

Serves: 4

Ingredients

Small Pack Cilantro (10g)

1 Lime

2 Large Avocados (400g), Stoned & Peeled

8 Whole Wheat Tortillas (330g)

10 Roasted Red Bell Peppers from a Jar

1/2 Cup (150g) Greek Yogurt

8 Cups Kale (130g)

14oz (400g) Can Chickpeas

2 Tsp Olive Oil

2 Tsp Ground Cumin

2 Tsp Smoked Paprika

1 Tsp Chili Powder

Method

1. Stone, peel and chop the avocados. Juice the lime. Chop the cilantro and roasted red peppers and shred the lettuce.

2. Heat oven to 425°F (220°C)/400°F (200°C) fan/gas 7. Drain the chickpeas and pour them in a large bowl. Add the olive oil, cumin, paprika and chili. Stir the chickpeas well to coat, then spread them onto a large baking tray and roast for 20-25 mins or until starting to crisp – give the tray a shake halfway through cooking to ensure they roast evenly. Remove from the oven and season to taste.

3. Toss the chopped avocados with the lime juice and chopped cilantro, then set aside until ready to serve.

4. Warm the tortillas following pack instructions, then pile in the avocado, kale, yogurt, peppers and toasted chickpeas at the table. Add more yogurt if needed to balance out the texture of the chickpeas and tortilla.

Spanish Sweet Potato Tortilla (Omelet)

Macronutrients & Omegas per Serving

Kcal:	624	Carbs:	50.7g	Vitamin C	31mg
Fat:	38.9g	Fiber:	8.9g	% of DV	34%
Protein:	20g	Cholesterol:	409mg		

A Spanish style tortilla filled with sweet potato and spinach that'll feed you and a partner for 2-3 lunches. Filled with spinach brimming with Vitamin C.

Benefits: Fiber, Prebiotics & Vitamin C

Value: $$

Time: 1 Hour 10

Serves: 4

Ingredients

2 Garlic Cloves, Thinly Sliced

2 Large Onions (275g), Thinly Sliced

4 Medium Sweet Potatoes, Thinly Sliced (1lb 12oz/800g)

8 Large Eggs (440g)

10 Cups (300g) Baby Spinach Leaves

8 Tbsp Olive Oil

Method

1. Heat 3 tbsp oil in a lidded large non-stick pan over a low-medium heat. Add the onions and cover for 15 mins, they should be soft but keep their color.

2. Boil some water. Add the spinach into a large colander and gently pour the boiling water all over it. Allow to cool, drain well and squeeze a little more water out of the spinach without crunching it too much. Separate any clumps gently.

3. Add 3 more tbsp oil, garlic and potatoes, season generously and mix thoroughly. Cover and cook for an additional 15 mins until the potatoes are very soft, stirring occasionally.

4. In a large bowl, whisk the eggs and add the cooked potato mixture, stirring thoroughly. Add the spinach and fold gently, keeping the soft potato intact.

5. Add 2 tbsp oil to the empty pan and pour back in the sweet potato egg mixture. Cover and cook the mixture over a low-medium heat for 20 mins. The base and sides should turn golden and the center should almost set. With a spatula, gently separate the sides from the pan to stop it from sticking.

6. Get a large plate, cover the tortilla and flip it. Return the tortilla back to the pan and cook for an additional 5 mins uncovered until the egg is fully set and its golden everywhere. If it breaks a little during the flip, it will set again in the final 5 mins of cooking. Use the spatula to separate the sides from the pan again.

7. Rest for 5 mins and then slide it onto a plate or board. Cut into wedges and serve.

Chicken, Spinach & Hummus Bowl

Macronutrients & Omegas per Serving

Kcal:	642	Carbs:		60.8g	Vitamin C	45mg
Fat:	26.6g	Fiber:		17g	% of DV	50%
Protein:	45.9g	Cholesterol:		77mg		

Another great dish for leftovers, quinoa and brown rice in particular. If you're feeling particularly artistic, keep all ingredients in each bowl separate and serve, allowing your guest the satisfaction of mixing everything together themself.

Benefits: Fiber, Prebiotics & Vitamin C

Value: $$

Time: 10 mins

Serves: 2

Ingredients

1/2 Red Onion (75g)

1 Small Lemon, Zested and Juiced

1 Small Avocado (100g), Stoned & Peeled

1 Cooked Chicken Breast (180g)

1/4 Cup (33g) Quinoa

1/3 Cup (33g) Brown Rice

1/2 Cup (100g) Pomegranate Seeds

1 1/4 Cups (200g) Hummus

6oz (170g) Baby Spinach

2 Tbsp Toasted Almonds

Method

1. Cook the quinoa and brown rice as per its instructions.

2. Chop the spinach, slice the avocado, finely slice the red onion and slice the chicken breast at an angle.

3. In a small bowl, add 2 tbsp hummus, half the lemon juice, all of the lemon zest and 1 tsp water. Mix thoroughly. The hummus should be of a consistency that allows it to be drizzled, but not too watery. Add additional water if need be.

4. In two bowls, evenly split the brown rice and quinoa. Add the hummus dressing and mix thoroughly. Top with spinach.

5. Squeeze the rest of the lemon juice over the avocado and add them to the bowl. Finally, add the chicken, pomegranate seeds, onion, almonds and remaining hummus. Mix both bowls thoroughly and serve.

Black-Eyed Pea Mole with Salsa

Macronutrients & Omegas per Serving

Kcal:	234	Carbs:		38.3g	Vitamin C	49mg
Fat:	6.3g	Fiber:		9.4g	% of DV	54%
Protein:	9g	Cholesterol:		0mg		

Home-made salsa and mole are an exceptional way to get some fresh vegetables and spices into your system. Onions, tomatoes and black-eyed peas are the key to adding fiber and prebiotics.

Benefits: Fiber, Prebiotics & Vitamin C

Value: $

Time: 25 mins

Serves: 2

Ingredients

1/2 Lime, Zest and Juice

1 Garlic Clove

2 Red Onion (300g)

2 Large Tomatoes (300g)

9oz (250g) Black-Eyed Peas

1/2 Tsp Ground Cinnamon

1 Tsp Vegetable Bouillon Powder

1 Tsp Ground Cilantro

1 Tsp Mild Chili Powder

2 Tsp Cocoa

2 Tsp Olive Oil

1 Tbsp Tomato Purée

2 Tbsp Fresh Cilantro

Method

1. Finely chop one red onion, halve and slice the other. Finely grate the garlic and chop both tomatoes.

2. Add the finely chopped red onion, tomatoes, 2 tbsp cilantro, lime zest and juice into a bowl and stir thoroughly.

3. In a non-stick pan heat 2 tsp olive oil. On a medium-high heat fry the onion and garlic until softened, stirring frequently. Add the rest of the cilantro, chili powder and ground cinnamon and stir thoroughly.

4. Add the can of black-eyed peas as well as their water, the cocoa, vegetable bouillon and tomato purée. Make sure the sauce becomes thick by stirring frequently.

5. Serve the mole into shallow bowls and top with your salsa.

Dinner

Chicken & Sweet Potato Curry

Macronutrients & Omegas per Serving

Kcal:	447	Carbs:		34.3g	Vitamin C	55mg
Fat:	23.9g	Fiber:		6.5g	% of DV	61%
Protein:	24g	Cholesterol:		118mg		

The curry paste can be swapped for any other kind, making this sweet potato curry customizable to your heat tolerance. A quick and easy mid-week meal.

Benefits: Prebiotics & Vitamin C
Value: $$
Time: 30 mins
Serves: 4

Ingredients

1 Green Chili Pepper Sweet or Spicy (45g)
1 Large Red Onion (185g)
2 Large Tomatoes (300g)
4 Sweet Potatoes (500g)
4 Skinless Chicken Thigh Fillets (480g)
4 Cups (120g) Spinach
1 Tbsp Olive Oil
2 Tbsp Rogan Josh Curry Paste

Method

1. Cut the sweet potato into 1-inch (2cm) cubes and the chicken and tomatoes into bite-sized pieces. Chop the tomatoes and peppers and cut the red onion into wedges.

2. Boil the sweet potatoes until tender for roughly 12 mins and then drain and set aside.

3. Heat 1 tbsp oil in a large frying pan and cook the chicken and onion together for 5 mins, until the chicken is cooked through. Add the curry paste and peppers, stir thoroughly and cook for 1 more min, add the tomatoes and cook for 1 last min.

4. Add 3fl oz (90ml) of boiling water to the frying pan and mix. Simmer for 5 mins then add the spinach and sweet potatoes and cook for an additional 2 mins. Serve either by itself or with brown rice.

Smoky Tomato & Bacon Spaghetti

Macronutrients & Omegas per Serving

Kcal:	560	Carbs:	85.3g	Vitamin C	12mg
Fat:	18.9g	Fiber:	12.4g	% of DV	13%
Protein:	20g	Cholesterol:	20mg		

Swapping regular spaghetti for a whole wheat version doubles the amount of fiber. This recipe contains a sneaky secret for thickening up sauces, add a ladle of pasta water!

Benefits: Fiber & Prebiotics

Value: $

Time: 25 mins

Serves: 4

Ingredients

1 Onion (110g)

2 Garlic Cloves

4 Slices (120g) Smoked Streaky Bacon

14oz (400g) Whole Wheat Spaghetti

2 X 14oz (400g) Cans Chopped Tomatoes

1 Tbsp Sweet Smoked Paprika

1 Tbsp Olive Oil

Method

1. Boil the spaghetti as per packet instructions. Slice the bacon into thin slices vertically and then into thirds horizontally. Finely chop the onion and garlic.

2. Heat 1 tbsp oil in a large non-stick pan and cook the bacon until it starts to crisp for 3-4 mins on a medium heat. Add the onion and cook for 4 mins then add the garlic and smoked paprika for 1 more min.

3. Pour in the chopped tomatoes and one ladle of pasta water, simmering for 5 mins until thick. Stir occasionally. Mix in the drained pasta and serve with grated cheese if you'd like.

Greek-Style Roast Fish

Macronutrients & Omegas per Serving

Kcal:	521	Carbs:	70.7g	Vitamin C	60mg
Fat:	16.1g	Fiber:	11.4g	% of DV	67%
Protein:	28.8g	Cholesterol:	71mg		

Although there are many great potatoes for roasting such as Yukon Gold or Maris Pipers, Russet potatoes come in at the higher spectrum of the fiber per potato ratio. Pollock or any other oily fish is a terrific addition to add some healthy fats.

Benefits: Fiber, Prebiotics & Vitamin C

Value: $$

Time: 1 Hour 10

Serves: 2

Ingredients

1/2 Lemon

Small Handful Parsley

2 Large Tomatoes (300g)

2 Fresh Pollock Fillets (200g)

2 Onions (220g)

3 Garlic Cloves, Roughly Chopped

3 Small Russet (or Maris Piper) Potatoes (500g)

1/2 Tsp Dried Oregano

2 Tbsp Olive Oil

Method

1. Preheat oven to 400°F (200°C)/350°F (180 °C) fan/gas 6. Scrub the potato then cut it into quarter wedges before parboiling them for 10 mins in salty water. Cut the lemon and tomatoes into wedges, halve and slice the onions then chop the garlic and parsley.

2. Add the parboiled potatoes, oregano and olive oil into a roasting tin, season, then mix together with your hands to coat everything in oil. Roast for 15 mins then turn everything over and add the onion and garlic, baking for 15 mins more.

3. Add the lemon and tomatoes and roast for 10 mins, then top with the fish fillets and cook for 10-12 mins until the fish is soft. Serve with parsley scattered over.

Chinese Curry Chicken

Macronutrients & Omegas per Serving

Kcal:	655	Carbs:		77.6g	Vitamin C	44mg
Fat:	17g	Fiber:		7.6g	% of DV	49%
Protein:	45.8g	Cholesterol:		110mg		

This recipe takes the "velveting" Chinese secret and makes it suitable for home-cooking. Velveting is the technique of coating chicken and quickly frying it to seal in its juices. The Chinese restaurant approach requires enough oil to fully submerge the chicken, so this recipe makes it home-cook friendly by switching that last step for blanching, i.e. parboiling the chicken.

Benefits: Prebiotics & Vitamin C

Value: $$

Time: 1 Hour

Serves: 4

Ingredients
Pinch Sugar
1 Onion (110g)
1 Garlic Clove
1 Green Chili Pepper Sweet or Spicy (45g)
2 Egg Whites (50g)
4 Skinless Chicken Breasts (600g)
2 Cups (320g) Frozen Peas
3 Cups (300g) Brown Rice
13.5floz (400ml) Chicken Stock
1/2 Tsp Ground Ginger
1 Tsp Turmeric
1 Tsp Soy Sauce
2 Tsp Salt
2 Tsp Curry Powder
2 Tbsp Cornstarch
3 Tbsp Olive Oil

Method

1. Cook the brown rice as per its instructions. Whisk the egg whites, cornstarch and salt in a bowl until smooth. Cut the chicken breasts into chunks and coat them in the marinade, marinating in the fridge for 30 mins.

2. Bring a pot of water to boil, add 1 tbsp olive oil and turn to a medium heat. Remove excess coating and add directly to boiling water for 1 min, just enough to keep the marinade coating intact, and then drain and set aside. The chicken should be opaque. It's ok if there are small clumps of egg white or cornstarch.

3. Dice the onion, crush the garlic and finely slice the pepper. Fry the onion in a wok on low to medium heat for 5 mins until they soften, then add the garlic and pepper and cook for 1 min. Stir in the spices and sugar and cook for another minute, add the stock and soy sauce, bring to a simmer and cook for 20 minutes. Tip everything into a blender and blend until smooth.

4. Fry the chicken in the remaining oil until it's browned all over. Tip the sauce back into the pan and bring everything to a simmer, stir in the peas and cook for 5 minutes. Add a little water if you need to thin the sauce. Serve with brown rice.

Pea, Paneer & Cauliflower Curry

Macronutrients & Omegas per Serving

Kcal:	484	Carbs:		57g	Vitamin C	110mg
Fat:	23.6g	Fiber:		12.8g	% of DV	122%
Protein:	17.8g	Cholesterol:		0mg		

The curry paste can be exchanged for one of your liking. The cauliflower, peas and naan give this recipe the kick of fiber it needs.

Benefits: Fiber, Prebiotics & Vitamin C

Value: $

Time: 1 Hour

Serves: 4

Ingredients

Small Pack (10g) Cilantro

1 Head (600g) of Cauliflower

2 Onions (220g)

2 Whole Wheat Naan (210g)

3 Garlic Cloves

2 Cups (250g) Paneer Cheese

7oz (200g) Frozen Peas

17.5oz (500g) Passata/Strained Tomatoes

2 Tbsp Olive Oil

2 Heaped Tbsp Tikka Masala Paste

Raita or Chutney, To Serve

Method

1. Chop the cauliflower into small pieces, cut the paneer cheese into medium-large cubes, thickly slice the onions, crush the garlic and chop the cilantro.

2. Heat 1 tbsp of oil in a large non-stick frying pan and fry the paneer cheese gently until crisp. Remove with a slotted spoon and set aside. Add the remaining oil and the cauliflower to the pan and cook until browned, roughly 10 mins for small pieces. Add the onions, and a little more oil if needed, and cook for a further 5 mins until softened. Stir in the garlic and curry paste, then pour in the passata, 8.5floz (250ml) water and add some seasoning. Bring to a simmer, then cover and cook for 18-20 mins or until the cauliflower is just tender. If the cauliflower wasn't cut small enough it may take additional time.

3. Add the frozen peas and crispy paneer to the pan and cook for a further 5 mins. Stir through most of the cilantro and garnish with the rest. Serve with naan bread and some minty raita or your favorite chutney.

Asparagus, Pea & Broad Bean Shakshuka

Macronutrients & Omegas per Serving

Kcal:	360	Carbs:	33.8g	Vitamin C	73mg
Fat:	17.9g	Fiber:	5.9g	% of DV	81%
Protein:	18.1g	Cholesterol:	207mg		

Shakshuka is a Middle Eastern and North African dish that combines tomatoes with spices and then poaches the eggs in the middle of this flavorful mixture. The whole wheat flatbread adds fiber, whilst the Greek yogurt adds probiotics.

Benefits: Prebiotics, Probiotics & Vitamin C

Value: $$

Time: 50 mins

Serves: 4

Ingredients

2 Scallions (30g)

4 Ripe Tomatoes (500g)

4 Large Eggs (220g)

4 Whole Wheat Flatbreads, To Serve

8 Asparagus Spears (125g)

1/3 Cup (50g) Peas

1/4 Cup (60g) Broad Beans

7oz (200g) Broccoli

2 Tbsp Olive Oil

2 Tbsp Chopped Parsley

4 Tbsp Greek Yogurt, To Serve

Large Pinch Cayenne Pepper, Plus Extra to Serve

Method

1. Remove the woody end of the asparagus then finely slice the spears, leaving 1-inch (2cm) intact at the top. Finely slice the broccoli, leaving the heads and 1-inch (2cm) of stalk intact. Finely slice the scallions then chop the tomatoes.

2. Heat the oil in a frying pan. Add the scallions, asparagus, broccoli, and fry gently until they soften a little, add the cumin seeds, cayenne, tomatoes (with their juices), parsley and plenty of seasoning, and stir. Cover with a lid and cook for 5 mins to make a base sauce, add the broccoli heads, cover and cook for an additional 2 mins. Add the asparagus spears, peas and broad beans, cover again and cook for 2 more mins.

3. Make 4 dips in the mixture. Break an egg into each dip, season well, cover with a lid and cook until the egg whites are just set. Serve with a spoonful of yogurt and some flatbreads, and sprinkle over another pinch of cayenne if you'd like.

Veggie Curry

Macronutrients & Omegas per Serving

Kcal:	622	Carbs:		112.3g	Vitamin C	56mg
Fat:	11.8g	Fiber:		17.8g	% of DV	62%
Protein:	21.4g	Cholesterol:		0mg		

Adding a curry spin to the chili con carne classic. This recipe is remarkably high in fiber and prebiotics thanks to the veg, beans and brown rice.

Benefits: Fiber, Prebiotics & Vitamin C

Value: $

Time: 35 mins

Serves: 2

Ingredients

(Optional) 1/2 Red Chili Pepper (23g)

Thumb-Sized Piece of Ginger (16g)

1 Onion (110g)

2 Garlic Cloves

2/3 Cup (10g) Cilantro, including Stalks and Leaves

1 1/2 Cup (150g) Brown Rice

14oz (400g) Can Chopped Tomatoes

14oz (400g) Can Kidney Beans

1 Tsp Ground Cumin

1 Tsp Ground Paprika

2 Tsp Curry Paste

1 Tbsp Olive Oil

Method

1. Cook the brown rice as per its instructions.

2. Peel the ginger and finely chop it alongside the onion, garlic and chili. Finely chop the cilantro stalks and shred its leaves.

3. Heat the oil in a large frying pan over a low-medium heat. Add the onion and a pinch of salt and cook slowly, stirring occasionally, until softened and just starting to color. Add the garlic, ginger and cilantro stalks and cook for a further 2 mins, until fragrant.

4. Add the spices to the pan and cook for another 1 min. Tip in the chopped tomatoes, kidney beans along with their water, and chili then bring to the boil.

5. Turn down the heat and simmer for 15 mins until the curry is nice and thick. Season to taste, then serve with the cooked brown rice and cilantro leaves.

Curried Cod

Macronutrients & Omegas per Serving

Kcal:	636	Carbs:	85.9g	Vitamin C	36mg
Fat:	16.2g	Fiber:	11.7g	% of DV	40%
Protein:	38.5g	Cholesterol:	70mg		

Trout has a very fishy taste which may not appeal to everyone's palate but fear not, a well-spiced curry can mask the flavor whilst maintaining the incredible amount of healthy fats.

Benefits: Fiber, Prebiotics & Vitamin C

Value: $$

Time: 35 mins

Serves: 4

Ingredients

Handful Cilantro

Thumb-Sized Piece Ginger (16g)

1/2 Red Chili Pepper (23g)

1 Onion (110g)

1 Lemon

4 Garlic Cloves

6 Skinless Trout Fillets (480g)

3 Cups (300g) Brown Rice

14oz (400g) Can Chickpeas

2 X 14oz (400g) Cans Chopped Tomatoes

1 Tbsp Olive Oil

2 Tbsp Medium Curry Powder

Method

1. Cook the brown rice as per its instructions.

2. Peel and finely grate the ginger, chop the onions and cilantro, crush the garlic, zest the lemon and then cut into wedges.

3. Heat the oil in a large, lidded frying pan. Cook the onion over a high heat for a few mins, then stir in the curry powder, ginger and garlic. Cook for another 1-2 mins until fragrant, then stir in the tomatoes, chickpeas and some seasoning.

4. Cook for 8-10 mins until thickened slightly, then top with the cod. Cover and cook for another 5-10 mins until the fish is cooked through. Scatter over the lemon zest and cilantro, then serve with the lemon wedges to squeeze over.

Roast Sea Bass with a Lemony Sweet Potato Salad

Macronutrients & Omegas per Serving

Kcal:	417	Carbs:	56.2g	Vitamin C	66mg
Fat:	8.6g	Fiber:	11.3g	% of DV	73%
Protein:	30.7g	Cholesterol:	53mg		

Another fish dish to keep your gut glad. Packed with Omega 3s from the sea bass as well as fiber and prebiotics from the sweet potatoes. Using the whole lemon, zest and juice, gives the dish a citrus twist.

Benefits: Fiber, Prebiotics & Vitamin C

Value: $$

Time: 1 hour 30 mins

Serves: 2

Ingredients

1 Lemon

1 Garlic Clove

2 Sea Bass Fillets (260g)

2 Large Sweet Potatoes (350g)

2 Red Onions (300g)

1/4 Cup (45g) Pomegranate Seeds

4.5oz (125g) Baby Spinach

1 Tsp Fennel Seeds

2 Tsp Extra Virgin Olive Oil

3 Tbsp Chopped Parsley

Method

1. Heat oven to 350°F (180°C)/325°F (160°C) fan/gas 4. Cut the red onions into wedges. Scrub the sweet potatoes and cut into cubes. Put in a roasting tin with the onions, fennel, and 6 whole garlic cloves, then toss with oil. Put the potatoes in the oven and roast for 25mins, turning everything over halfway through.

2. Zest the whole lemon and then slice it in half. Cut one half into rounds. Put the fish fillets on top of the roasted potatoes and place the lemon rounds on the fish. Roast for 5 mins.

3. Finely chop the garlic. Squeeze the other half of the lemon into a bowl and mix it with the lemon zest, parsley, garlic, oil and some black pepper.

4. Remove the potatoes and fish from the oven. Temporarily take the fish off, stir in the spinach and add the fillets back on top. Roast for 2 more mins.

5. Remove the fish and potatoes from the oven. Place one sea bass fillet on each plate. Add the lemon mixture and pomegranate seeds to the potatoes, spinach and onions and toss thoroughly. Serve the salad, placing the fillets to one side or on top.

Grilled Tuna Steaks with Quinoa Salad & Mint Chutney

Macronutrients & Omegas per Serving

Kcal:	338	Carbs:		38.1g	Vitamin C	44mg
Fat:	9g	Fiber:		6.6g	% of DV	49%
Protein:	27.6g	Cholesterol:		32mg		

A minty yogurt marinade transforms delicious tuna steaks into a probiotic contender not to be messed with! Accompanied by some vegetables and quinoa for the much-needed fiber.

Benefits: Prebiotics, Probiotics & Vitamin C

Value: $$$

Time: 30 mins

Serves: 2

Ingredients

1/4 Cucumber (75g)

Good Squeeze of Lemon Juice

Pinch of Cumin Seeds

1 Garlic Clove

1 Small Red Onion (100g)

4 Tomatoes (500g)

1/3 Cup (60g) Quinoa

1/2 Cup (150g) Greek Yogurt

4 X 4oz (115g) Thin Tuna Steaks

1/4 Tsp Turmeric

3 Tbsp Chopped Mint

3 Tbsp Chopped Cilantro

Method

1. Put 2 tbsp of the mint and cilantro in a bowl. Add the yogurt and garlic, and blitz with a hand blender until smooth. Stir 2 tbsp of the herby yogurt with the turmeric and cumin, then add the fish and turn in the mixture to completely coat. Marinate in a closed bag for at least 15 mins, preferably an hour.

2. Boil the quinoa as per its instructions. Drain well.

3. Chop the mint, cilantro, and tomatoes. Finely chop the red onion and finely dice the cucumber.

4. Preheat the oven broiler/grill to high. If placing the fish on a grill grate, lightly oil the grate first. Arrange the fish in a shallow heatproof dish and grill for 5-7 mins per side, depending on thickness, until it flakes.

5. Toss the quinoa with the cucumber, onion, tomatoes, lemon juice and remaining herbs. Spoon onto a plate, add the fish and spoon round the mint chutney, or add it at the table.

Garlic Turkey Meatballs with Vegetable Sauce

Macronutrients & Omegas per Serving

Kcal:	595	Carbs:	78.6g	Vitamin C	85mg
Fat:	18.1g	Fiber:	33.1g	% of DV	94%
Protein:	40.9g	Cholesterol:	57mg		

Turkey is a leaner counterpart to its chicken rival but is ideal for poultry meatballs! A wholesome vegetable dish at its heart with plenty of flavor.

Benefits: Fiber, Prebiotics & Vitamin C

Value: $$

Time: 1 Hour

Serves: 4

Ingredients

1 Onion (110g)

1 Fennel Bulb (234g)

1 Broccoli (150g)

2 Carrots (120g)

2 Celery Sticks (80g)

3 Garlic Cloves

14oz (400g) Lean Ground Turkey Breast

17.5oz (500g) Passata/Strained Tomatoes

1.5lb (700g) New/Baby Potatoes

17floz (500ml) Chicken Stock

1 Tsp Fennel Seed

2 Tbsp Chopped Parsley

2 Tbsp Olive Oil

4 Tbsp (22g) Oats

Method

1. Finely chop the onion and 2 garlic cloves then finely dice the carrots and celery. Halve the fennel bulb and thinly slice, keeping the fronds (feathery leaves at the top). Crush the teaspoon of fennel seeds and 1 garlic. Chop the broccoli into bite-sized pieces and remove the hard part of the stalk.

2. Heat 1 tbsp oil in a large non-stick frying pan with a lid, then tip in the onion, carrots, celery, garlic and fennel, and stir well. Cover the pan and cook over a medium heat for 8 mins, stirring every now and then. Pour in the passata/strained tomatoes and stock, cover and leave to simmer for 20 mins.

3. Place the new/baby potatoes in a pan of boiling water and gently simmer for 15-20 mins until tender.

4. Tip the ground meat into a large bowl. Add the oats, fennel seeds and leaves, the garlic and plenty of black pepper, and mix in with your hands. Shape into 25 meatballs about the size of a walnut. Heat 1 tbsp olive oil in a non-stick pan and gently cook the meatballs until they take on a little color. Give the sauce a stir, then add the meatballs and parsley. Cover and cook for 3 mins, then add the broccoli and cook for another 7 mins until the meatballs are cooked through and the veg in the sauce is tender.

5. Serve together with the drained potatoes, adding a little butter if you desire.

Layered Eggplant & Lentil Bake

Macronutrients & Omegas per Serving

Kcal:	456	Carbs:	57.4g	Vitamin C	36mg
Fat:	18.7g	Fiber:	14.3g	% of DV	40%
Protein:	21g	Cholesterol:	25mg		

A fibrous vegetarian style meal that contains a large amount of protein from its lentils. The mozzarella can be exchanged for a nut or soy-based cheese to make the recipe vegan friendly.

Benefits: Fiber, Prebiotics, Probiotics & Vitamin C

Value: $

Time: 1 hour

Serves: 4

Ingredients

Small Pack (5g) Basil Leaves

2 Eggplant (800g)

2 Onions (220g)

3 Garlic Cloves

3/4 Cup (145g) Green Lentils

2 Cups Butternut Squash Cubes (300g)

4.5oz (125g) Mozzarella Ball

14oz (400g) Can Chopped Tomatoes

3 Tbsp Olive Oil

Method

1. Cut eggplant into 1/4-inch (0.5 cm) slices lengthways. Finely chop the onions and garlic and dice the butternut squash.

2. Heat oven to 425°F (220°C)/400°F (200°C) fan/gas 7. Brush both sides of the eggplant with 2 tbsp olive oil and lay alongside the squash on baking sheets. Season and bake for 15-20 mins until tender, turning once.

3. Cook the lentils following its instructions.

4. Heat the remaining oil in a large frying pan. Tip in the onions and garlic and cook until soft. Add the tomatoes, plus ½ can of water. Simmer for 10-15 mins until the sauce has thickened. Stir in the lentils, basil and seasoning.

5. Spoon a layer of lentils into a small baking dish. Top with eggplant slices, then lentils and repeat, finishing with a layer of eggplant. Scatter with torn mozzarella pieces and bake for a further 15 mins until the cheese is golden and bubbling.

Tomato, Sweet Potato & Zucchini Stew

Macronutrients & Omegas per Serving

Kcal:	267	Carbs:	48.5g	Vitamin C	42mg
Fat:	6.1g	Fiber:	8.8g	% of DV	47%
Protein:	8.2g	Cholesterol:	5mg		

A low-calorie starter dish that can double a main course if there's any remaining leftover meat or beans, just throw them in the stew alongside the tomatoes! Contains a good macronutrient split across the board.

Benefits: Fiber, Prebiotics & Vitamin C

Value: $

Time: 1 Hour 10 mins

Serves: 4

Ingredients

Small Bunch Basil (5g)

1 Onion (110g)

2 Garlic Cloves

3 Zucchinis (588g)

4 Large Sweet Potatoes (650g)

2 X 14oz (400g) Cans Chopped Tomatoes

1 Tbsp Olive Oil

5 Tbsp (25g) Parmesan

Method

1. Quarter the zucchinis lengthways and then cut into chunks. Chop the onion, crush the garlic and cut the sweet potatoes into chunks. Tear the basil and finely grate the parmesan.

2. Heat the oil in a large frying pan over a medium heat. Add the onion and cook for about 10 mins until softened and starting to go golden brown. Add the garlic and cook for 5 mins more.

3. Add the zucchinis and cook for about 5 mins until starting to soften. Tip in the tomatoes and give everything a good stir. Simmer for 20 mins, then add the sweet potatoes and simmer for an additional 15-20 mins or until tomatoes are reduced and the zucchinis and potatoes are soft, then stir in the basil and Parmesan. Serve.

Mexican Penne with Avocado

Macronutrients & Omegas per Serving

Kcal:	370	Carbs:	60.3g	Vitamin C	68mg
Fat:	11.2g	Fiber:	14.5g	% of DV	76%
Protein:	13.9g	Cholesterol:	1mg		

A spicy pasta dish that can be tailored to your taste buds. Turn down the heat by switching the hot chili powder to medium, excluding the jalapeno and adding additional yogurt. Add more whole wheat pasta if you'd like leftovers.

Benefits: Fiber, Prebiotics, Probiotics & Vitamin C

Value: $

Time: 30 mins

Serves: 4

Ingredients

1/2 Jalapeno Pepper
1/2 Lime
Handful Cilantro
1 Large Onion (140g)
1 Orange Bell Pepper (120g)
1 Avocado (200g)
2 Garlic Cloves
1 1/2 Cups (150g) Whole Wheat Penne
14oz (400g) Can Chopped Tomatoes
14oz (400g) Can Lima Beans
½ Tsp Cumin Seeds
1 Tsp Olive Oil
1 Tsp Ground Cilantro
1 Tsp Vegetable Bouillon Powder
2 Tsp Hot Chili Powder
2 Tbsp Greek Yogurt

Method

1. Finely chop 1 tbsp onion and then slice the rest. Deseed and cut the orange bell pepper into chunks. Slice the jalapeno (if using), grate the garlic, zest and juice 1/2 lime, stone, peel and chop the avocado and chop the cilantro.

2. Heat the oil in a medium pan. Add the sliced onion and pepper and fry, stirring frequently for 10 mins until golden. Stir in the garlic and spices, then tip in the tomatoes, half a can of water, the corn and bouillon. Cover and simmer for 15 mins.

3. Cook the pasta as per its instructions until al dente.

4. Meanwhile, toss the avocado with the lime juice and zest, and the finely chopped onion.

5. Drain the penne and toss into the sauce with the cilantro. Spoon the pasta into bowls, top with the avocado and jalapeno slices, scatter over the cilantro leaves and a dollop of Greek yogurt.

Spicy Roast Veg & Lentils

Macronutrients & Omegas per Serving

Kcal:	678	Carbs:	106.2g	Vitamin C	170mg
Fat:	13.4g	Fiber:	24.9g	% of DV	189%
Protein:	42.5g	Cholesterol:	0mg		

Roasted vegetable dishes require lots of prep work, and then the challenging work pays off when you throw it in the oven and relax. All of the veg and beans culminate into a very fibrous meal.

Benefits: Fiber, Prebiotics & Vitamin C

Value: $

Time: 1 hour

Serves: 4

Ingredients

1 Red Onion (150g)

1 Small-Medium Butternut Squash (1lb/950g)

Large Handful Cilantro

2 Garlic Cloves

3 Bell Peppers (360g)

21oz (600g) Can Puy Lentils

5floz (150ml) Hot Vegetable Stock

3 Tbsp Olive Oil

3 Tbsp Curry Paste

Method

1. Using a sharp knife, peel the butternut squash. Cut it in half lengthways, scoop out the seeds, then cut into small-medium cubes. Halve and thickly slice the onion, deseed and cut the bell peppers into 0.5-inch (1cm) wide strips. Drain and rinse the lentils. Chop the cilantro and finely chop the garlic.

2. Heat oven to 400°F (200°C)/350°F (180°C) fan/gas 6. Put the squash cubes in a large roasting tin with the onion, and garlic. Mix the oil with curry paste and drizzle over the vegetables. Toss well to coat in the curry mix and season.

3. Roast for 20 mins then add the peppers and roast for an additional 10 mins until the vegetables are beginning to soften.

4. Make the vegetable stock as per instructions or heat pre-made stock. Add the lentils and stock to the roasting tin and mix. Return to the oven for a further 5-10 mins until the vegetables are tender. Stir in the cilantro and serve immediately.

Prawn Jalfrezi

Macronutrients & Omegas per Serving

Kcal:	572	Carbs:		102.2g	Vitamin C	133mg
Fat:	9.6g	Fiber:		11.7g	% of DV	148%
Protein:	24.8g	Cholesterol:		2mg		

Nothing beats giant juicy prawns in a Jalfrezi. This humble Indian dish is greater than the sum of its parts, showcasing how the right mixture of spices create an aromatic sauce. If the sauce is too thick for your liking, add a few tablespoons of water.

Benefits: Fiber, Prebiotics, Probiotics & Vitamin C

Value: $$$

Time: 35 mins

Serves: 2

Ingredients

1/2 Lemon

Small Bunch Cilantro

Thumb-Sized Piece Ginger (16g)

1 Large Green Bell Pepper (150g)

2 Onions (220g)

2 Garlic Cloves

8 Tiger Prawns (140g)

1 1/2 Cups Brown Rice (150g)

14oz (400g) Can Chopped Tomato

¼ Tsp Chili Flakes

½ Tsp Ground Turmeric

½ Tsp Ground Cumin

1 Tsp Ground Cilantro

2 Tsp Olive Oil

1 Tbsp Curry Paste

1 Tbsp Clear Honey

2 Tbsp Greek Yogurt

Method

1. Chop the onions and garlic then finely chop the ginger. Halve, deseed and chop the green bell pepper. Separate the stalks from the leaves of the cilantro and chop both. Squeeze the lemon juice into a bowl. Peel and clean the prawns. Cook the brown rice as per its instructions.

2. Heat the oil in a non-stick pan and fry the onions, ginger and garlic for 6 mins, stirring frequently, until softened and starting to color. If you've bought the prawns pre-cooked, skip this step and continue cooking the onions for 2 more mins, otherwise add the uncooked prawns, cook for an additional 2 mins then remove the prawns and set aside.

3. Add the spices and chili flakes, stir briefly, then pour in the tomatoes with the honey. Stir in the pepper, cilantro stalks and prawns. Cover the pan and leave to simmer for 5 mins, then add the prawns and simmer for an additional 5 mins. The mixture will be very thick and splutter a little, so stir frequently. The shrimps are cooked when they've shrunk in size and are no long shrinking, exterior is pink and flesh slightly white in color. If the flesh is bright white, the shrimps may be overcooked.

4. Scatter over the cilantro leaves. Serve the rice and prawn jalfrezi with Greek yogurt if you'd like.

Miso Brown Rice & Chicken Salad

Macronutrients & Omegas per Serving

Kcal:	588	Carbs:	78.2g	Vitamin C	68mg
Fat:	10.7g	Fiber:	14.9g	% of DV	76%
Protein:	44.8g	Cholesterol:	110mg		

Capitalizing on miso's probiotic profile, this quick rice dish provides an influx of healthy bacteria directly to the gut.

Benefits: Fiber, Probiotics & Vitamin C

Value: $$

Time: 45 mins

Serves: 2

Ingredients

2 Skinless Chicken Breasts (300g)

4 Scallions (60g)

1 1/2 Cups (150g) Brown Basmati Rice

5oz (140g) Sprouting Broccoli

2 Tsp Grated Ginger

4 Tsp Miso Paste

1 Tbsp Toasted Sesame Seeds

2 Tbsp Rice Vinegar

2 Tbsp Mirin

Method

1. Cook the rice as per its instructions then drain and keep warm. Cut the onions into diagonal slices.

2. Place the chicken breasts into a pan of boiling water so they are completely covered. Boil for 1 min, then turn off the heat, place a lid on and let it sit for 15 mins. When cooked through, cut into slices.

3. Boil the broccoli until tender. Drain, rinse under cold water and drain again.

4. For the dressing, mix the miso, rice vinegar, mirin and ginger together.

5. Divide the rice between two plates and scatter over the scallions and sesame seeds. Place the broccoli and chicken slices on top. To finish, drizzle over the dressing.

Barbequed Sweet Potatoes Filled with a Chickpea Spinach Salad

Macronutrients & Omegas per Serving

Kcal:	467	Carbs:	52.4g	Vitamin C	21mg
Fat:	25.4g	Fiber:	11.8g	% of DV	23%
Protein:	12.2g	Cholesterol:	2mg		

Time for a summer sweet potato treat! This dish has multiple levels of flavor: crispy potato skin, sweet potato, sour Greek yogurt tahini and juicy pomegranate seeds.

Benefits: Fiber, Prebiotics & Probiotics

Value: $

Time: 1 hour 20

Serves: 4

Ingredients

Small Bunch Dill (5g)

1 Large Garlic Clove

1 Echalion Shallot (50g)

1 Lemon

4 Medium Sweet Potatoes (520g)

1/4 Cup (25g) Toasted Walnuts

2/3 Cup (110g) Pomegranate Seeds

2 1/2 Cups (75g) Baby Leaf Spinach

14oz (400g) Can Chickpeas

2 Tbsp Tahini

3 1/2 Tbsp Greek Yogurt

4 Tbsp Olive Oil

Method

1. Crush the garlic and finely chop the shallot and dill. Zest and Juice the lemon then drain the chickpeas.

2. Wrap each potato in foil and put directly on the hot coals of a barbecue for 35-45 mins, depending on the size of the potatoes. Insert a skewer into each one to check that they're cooked. Alternatively, heat oven to 400°F (200°C)/350°F (180°C) fan/gas 6 and put the foil-wrapped potatoes on a large baking sheet. Bake in the oven for 45 mins-1 hour or until the center is soft. Once cooked, put under a hot grill for 3 mins until the skin is blackened and crispy.

3. After 20 mins of barbecuing the potatoes (or 35 mins of baking them), heat 1 tbsp olive oil in a large frying pan over a medium heat. Add the garlic and shallot and fry for 2-3 mins until softened, then stir the chickpeas into the mixture. Gently warm for 1 min, add the spinach and leave to wilt. Add the dill.

4. Whisk together the lemon juice, zest and 3 tbsp olive oil in a small bowl. Season to taste and stir into the chickpea mixture. Gently mash with a potato masher until the chickpeas are slightly crushed. Mix together the yogurt and tahini in another small bowl, and season to taste with salt.

5. Split the potatoes open lengthways. Fill with the bean mixture, drizzle over the tahini yogurt and top with the hazelnuts and pomegranate seeds.

Butternut Squash Casserole

Macronutrients & Omegas per Serving

Kcal:	343	Carbs:		61.7g	Vitamin C	81mg
Fat:	9.3g	Fiber:		11.5g	% of DV	90%
Protein:	9.6g	Cholesterol:		2mg		

An easy casserole that requires plenty of up-front preparation, then sitting back and relaxing once it's in the oven. Perfect for scaling to larger batches. Feel free to add additional chili powder to increase the heat or offset the heat with more yogurt.

Benefits: Fiber, Prebiotics, Probiotics & Vitamin C

Value: $$

Time: 1 Hour

Serves: 4

Ingredients

1 Onion (110g)
1 Red Bell Pepper (120g)
1 Butternut Squash (550g)
2 Garlic Cloves
2 Sweet Potatoes (260g)
1/2 Cup (90g) Bulgur Wheat
14oz (400g) Can Chopped Tomato
17floz (500ml) Vegetable Stock
1 Tsp Cumin Seeds
2 Tbsp Olive Oil
2 Tbsp Paprika
4 Tbsp Greek Yogurt

Method

1. Slice the onion, crush the garlic, deseed and chop the bell pepper, peel the squash and then chop both the squash and sweet potatoes into small cubes.

2. In a large pan, heat the olive oil, then cook the onion and garlic for 5-7 mins until the onion is softened. Add the cumin seeds and paprika, then cook for a further 2 mins. Stir in the sweet potato, red bell pepper and butternut squash and toss with the onion and spices for 2 mins.

3. Pour in the tomatoes, vegetable stock, season, then simmer gently for 15 mins. Stir in the bulgur wheat, cover with a lid, then simmer for 15 mins more until the sweet potato and squash are tender, the bulgur wheat is cooked, and the liquid has been absorbed.

4. Serve in bowls topped with a spoonful of Greek yogurt.

Pumpkin and Chickpea Curry

Macronutrients & Omegas per Serving

Kcal:	575	Carbs:		66.8g	Vitamin C	38mg
Fat:	32g	Fiber:		11g	% of DV	42%
Protein:	15.8g	Cholesterol:		0mg		

Complemented by the coconut milk and assortment of spices, Thai curry paste adds a heap of flavor. If you don't have naan bread, substitute it with 3/4 cup of brown rice per person.

Benefits: Fiber, Prebiotics & Vitamin C

Value: $

Time: 40 mins

Serves: 4

Ingredients

Large Handful Mint Leaves

1 Piece Pumpkin or Small Squash (35oz/1kg)

2 Whole Wheat Naan Bread (212g)

2 Limes

2 Onions (220g)

2 Large Stalks Lemongrass

6 Cardamom Pods

14oz (400g) Can Chickpeas

13.5floz (400ml) Can Coconut Milk

1/2 Tsp Chili Flakes

1 Tbsp Olive Oil

1 Tbsp Mustard Seed

3 Tbsp Yellow Thai Curry Paste

Method

1. Finely chop the onions and bash the lemongrass with the back of a knife. Drain and rinse the chickpeas. Dice the pumpkin or squash into small cubes.

2. Heat the oil in a sauté pan, then gently fry the curry paste with the onions, lemongrass, cardamom, chili flakes and mustard seed for 2-3 mins until fragrant. Stir the pumpkin or squash into the pan and coat in the paste, then pour in the stock and coconut milk. Bring everything to a simmer, add the chickpeas, then cook for about 10 mins until the pumpkin is tender, if using butternut squash this could take 15 mins depending on how small the cubes are.

3. Squeeze the juice of one lime into the curry, then cut the other lime into wedges to serve alongside. Just before serving, remove the lemongrass and tear over mint leaves, then bring to the table with lime wedges and warm naan breads.

Teriyaki Salmon with Pak Choi

Macronutrients & Omegas per Serving

Kcal:	662	Carbs:	78.9g	Vitamin C	58mg
Fat:	23.2g	Fiber:	8.1g	% of DV	64%
Protein:	35g	Cholesterol:	72mg		

A succulent salmon fillet bathed in a teriyaki style sauce with one major change, no sesame oil, as it contains a moderate quantity of unhealthy fats (Omega 6). This recipe goes to show that you can make simple substitutions that have minor impact on flavor but substantial impact on health.

Benefits: Fiber, Prebiotics & Vitamin C

Value: $$$

Time: 30 mins

Serves: 2

Ingredients

2 Skinless Salmon Fillets (260g)

3 Garlic Cloves

1 1/2 Cups (150g) Brown Rice

9oz (250g) Bok Choy

2 Tsp Grated Ginger

5 Tsp Olive Oil

1 Tbsp Sweet Chili Sauce

1 Tbsp Honey

1 Tbsp Mirin

2 Tbsp Soy Sauce

Method

1. Grate the ginger and garlic.

2. Heat the oven to 400°F (200°C)/350°F (180°C) fan/gas 6 and put 2 skinless salmon fillets in a shallow baking dish. Cook the brown rice as per its instructions.

3. Mix 1 tbsp sweet chili sauce, 1 tbsp honey, 1 tsp olive oil, 1 tbsp mirin or dry sherry, 2 tbsp soy sauce and 2 tsp finely grated ginger in a small bowl and pour over the salmon so the fillets are completely covered. Bake for 15-20 mins. To test if done, put a toothpick through the thickest part, if you feel resistance then it's still raw, if you feel no resistance then it's done.

4. Cut a slice across the base of 2 large bok choy so the leaves separate. Heat 4 tsp olive oil in a wok, add 3 grated garlic cloves and stir-fry briefly to soften, then add the bok choy and fry for 1-2 mins.

5. Serve the bok choy in shallow bowls, top with salmon and spoon over the juices. Serve with brown rice.

Ground Beef & Sweet Potato Stew

Macronutrients & Omegas per Serving

Kcal:	496	Carbs:		41.4g	Vitamin C	57mg
Fat:	26.6g	Fiber:		8g	% of DV	63%
Protein:	24.1g	Cholesterol:		80mg		

A hearty winter stew which is perfect for scaling up and freezing. Sweet potato brings the fiber and the Worcestershire sauce adds the tang.

Benefits: Fiber, Prebiotics & Vitamin C

Value: $$

Time: 1 hour 20

Serves: 4

Ingredients

Few Thyme Sprigs
Handful Parsley
2 Onions (220g)
2 Carrots (120g)
1 Celery Stick (50g)
1 Bell Pepper (120g)
1 Beef Bouillon Cube
1 Bay Leaf
14oz (400g) Can Chopped Tomato
1lb (450g) Ground Beef
1lb (450g) Sweet Potatoes
1 Tbsp Olive Oil
1 Tbsp Tomato Purée
1 Tbsp Worcestershire Sauce

Method

1. Roughly chop the onions, carrots, bell pepper and parsley, slice the celery stick. Cut the sweet potato into large chunks.

2. Heat the oil in a large pan, add the onion, carrot and celery, and cook on low heat for 10 mins, stirring frequently until soft. Add the beef and cook until it's browned all over.

3. Add the tomato purée and cook for a few mins, then add the Worcestershire sauce, tomatoes, sweet potatoes, bell pepper, herbs, can full of water and bouillon cube. Bring to the boil.

4. Simmer on a low heat for 40-45 mins until the sweet potatoes are tender, stirring a few times throughout cooking to make sure they are cooking evenly.

5. Once cooked, remove the bay leaf, stir through the chopped parsley and serve with cabbage.

Conclusion

If you or someone close to you is suffering from peptic ulcer disease it can be emotionally and physically damaging. However, you are not alone. As science progresses, we are gaining new insights, allowing us to fully understand the mechanisms behind peptic ulcer disease and how to support its healing process.

The amount of people that will develop peptic ulcers in their lifetime is astonishing. Luckily for us, this disease is curable with the help of a physician. There are also numerous methods of supporting the healing process or alleviating symptoms that can be implemented from your very home. Increasing prebiotic, probiotic and vitamin C intake can promote the beneficial effects of a healthy bacterial ecosystem as well as decreasing the side-effects from taking antibiotics.

As digestive disorders are becoming more frequent, the attention from the medical community similarly rises. So, I urge you to take your health seriously, consult a physician, adopt lifestyle changes and focus on your eating habits. Most people with peptic ulcers will never experience serious complications. Hopefully, we'll keep it that way. As time presses forwards, we're likely to learn more but, in the meantime, I wish you good health.

Appendix

How Stomach Acid is Produced

Gastric acid secretion is regulated by specific hormones, particularly gastrin, and the nervous system via the vagus nerve, which runs from the face through to the abdomen. Gastrin is a hormone that plays a leading role in stimulating the production of gastric acid and is produced by glands in the pyloric antrum region of the stomach, which can be seen in figure 3 on the next page. Gastrin is released in response to various stimuli, such as the presence of partially digested proteins in the gastrointestinal tract and even from laying your eyes on a mouth-watering burger[56].

The gastric acid that's produced by the stomach is hydrochloric acid (chemical sign HCl) and is extremely potent, with a pH of 1 it's 10 times more acidic than lemon juice. The pH scale starts from most acidic at 0, becomes neutral at 7, then most alkaline at 14. Gastric acid excels in performing its vital function, breaking down food to allow the body to fully absorb nutrients. In fact, gastric acid is so potent that a complex protection mechanism is invoked every time the acid is produced. If a peptic ulcer is present along the lining of the stomach or duodenum, then any contact with this acid can exacerbate the problem whilst preventing it from healing.

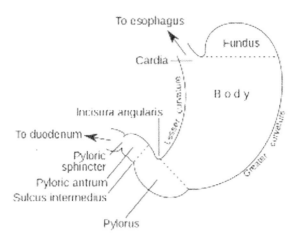

Figure 3 - Sections of the Human Stomach – Author Henry Vandyke Carter, under Public domain.

Cells from the inner cell layer of the fundus and cardia secrete this hydrochloric acid. These cells perform the following complex steps simultaneously, they are not in order:

1. Water (H_2O) reacts with carbon dioxide (CO_2) within the parietal cell to form carbonic acid (H_2CO_3) which separates into hydrogen ions H^+ and bicarbonate ions HCO_3^-

2. Potassium ions (K^+) disperse into the stomach (aka gastric lumen in the picture below)

3. The **proton pump** then exchanges K^+ in the stomach for H^+

4. Chloride ions (Cl^-) disperse passively into the stomach, their negative charge balancing the positive charge of the H^+ which means the stomach now contains **HCl**, or hydrochloric acid.

5. The parietal cells import Cl^- from the blood to counteract losing them in the stomach, HCO_3^- are exchanged in the process

The gastric acid, or hydrochloric acid (HCl), therefore, comes from the combination of H^+ from water and Cl^- from blood.

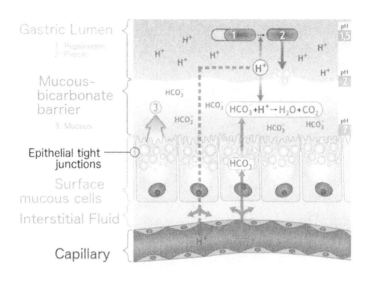

Figure 4 - Gastric Mucosal Barrier – Author Nelson Glyn, under Creative Commons BY-SA (https://creativecommons.org/licenses/by-sa/4.0), made grayscale.

Protection from Stomach Acid

As you can see from the diagram above, due to the hydrogen ions and chloride ions only combining once they meet in the gastric lumen, the pH level of the parietal cells remains a neutral 7. This is the first defensive mechanism.

The second layer of defense is a thick coat of mucous called the mucous-bicarbonate barrier which covers the entire surface of the stomach lining. It's excreted from mucous cells (goblet cells) and prevents acid and enzymes from reaching the wall lining. HCO_3^- is trapped within the mucous which can neutralize any HCl that manages to enter it.

The final wall of defense is the epithelial tight junctions. These are a compact lining of cells which can repel harsh fluids from entering. Once food is broken down by the gastric acid and enzymes mixture, it's ready to be passed into the small intestine. The acidity is then neutralized rapidly by HCO_3^- produced by the pancreas.

Sources

[1] Aro, Pertti, Tom Storskrubb, Jukka Ronkainen, Elisabeth Bolling-Sternevald, Lars Engstrand, Michael Vieth, Manfred Stolte, Nicholas J. Talley, and Lars Agréus. "Peptic ulcer disease in a general adult population: the Kalixanda study: a random population-based study." American journal of epidemiology 163, no. 11 (2006): 1025-1034.

[2] Yeomans, Neville D., and Jorgen Naesdal. "Systematic review: ulcer definition in NSAID ulcer prevention trials." *Alimentary pharmacology & therapeutics* 27, no. 6 (2008): 465-472.

[3] Fink, G. "Stress controversies: post-traumatic stress disorder, hippocampal volume, gastroduodenal ulceration." Journal of neuroendocrinology 23, no. 2 (2011): 107-117.

[4] Ryan-Harshman, Milly, and Walid Aldoori. "How diet and lifestyle affect duodenal ulcers. Review of the evidence." Canadian family physician 50, no. 5 (2004): 727-732.

[5] Warren, J. Robin, and Barry Marshall. "Unidentified curved bacilli on gastric epithelium in active chronic gastritis." The lancet 321, no. 8336 (1983): 1273-1275.

[6] Watts, Geoff. "Nobel prize is awarded to doctors who discovered H pylori." (2005): 795.

[7] Ramakrishnan, Kalyanakrishnan, and Robert C. Salinas. "Peptic ulcer disease." *American family physician* 76, no. 7 (2007): 1005-1012.

[8] Berg, Gabriele, Günter Bode, Maria Blettner, Heiner Boeing, and Hermann Brenner. "Helicobacter pylori infection and serum ferritin: A population-based study among 1806 adults in Germany." The American journal of gastroenterology 96, no. 4 (2001): 1014-1018.

[9] Maekita, Takao, Kazuyuki Nakazawa, Mami Mihara, Takeshi Nakajima, Kimihiko Yanaoka, Mikitaka Iguchi, Kenji Arii et al. "High levels of aberrant DNA methylation in Helicobacter pylori–infected gastric mucosae and its possible association with gastric cancer risk." Clinical Cancer Research 12, no. 3 (2006): 989-995.

[10] Muhammad, Jibran Sualeh, Mohamed Ahmed Eladl, and Ghalia Khoder. "Helicobacter pylori-induced DNA methylation as an epigenetic modulator of gastric cancer: recent outcomes and future direction." Pathogens 8, no. 1 (2019): 23.

[11] Blaser, Martin J. "Helicobacter pylori and the pathogenesis of gastroduodenal inflammation." Journal of Infectious Diseases 161, no. 4 (1990): 626-633.

[12] Yamaoka, Yoshio, ed. Helicobacter pylori: molecular genetics and cellular biology. Horizon Scientific Press, 2008.

[13] Kusters, Johannes G., Arnoud HM van Vliet, and Ernst J. Kuipers. "Pathogenesis of Helicobacter pylori infection." Clinical microbiology reviews 19, no. 3 (2006): 449-490.

[14] Huang, Jia-Qing, Subbaramiah Sridhar, and Richard H. Hunt. "Role of Helicobacter pylori infection and non-steroidal anti-inflammatory drugs in peptic-ulcer disease: a meta-analysis." The Lancet 359, no. 9300 (2002): 14-22.

[15] Rostom, Alaa, Catherine Dube, George A. Wells, Peter Tugwell, Vivian Welch, Emilie Jolicoeur, Jessie McGowan, and Angel Lanas. "Prevention of NSAID-induced gastroduodenal ulcers." Cochrane database of systematic reviews 4 (2002).

[16] Laporte, Joan-Ramon, Luisa Ibanez, Xavier Vidal, Lourdes Vendrell, and Roberto Leone. "Upper gastrointestinal bleeding associated with the use of NSAIDs." Drug safety 27, no. 6 (2004): 411-420.

[17] Ko, J. K., and C. H. Cho. "Alcohol drinking and cigarette smoking: a" partner" for gastric ulceration." Zhonghua yi xue za zhi= Chinese medical journal; Free China ed 63, no. 12 (2000): 845-854.

[18] Ma, Li, Jimmy YC Chow, and Chi H. Cho. "Effects of cigarette smoking on gastric ulcer formation and healing: possible mechanisms of action." Journal of clinical gastroenterology 27 (1998): S80-S86.

[19] Svanes, C., J. A. Søreide, A. Skarstein, B. T. Fevang, P. Bakke, S. E. Vollset, K. Svanes, and O. Søreide. "Smoking and ulcer perforation." Gut 41, no. 2 (1997): 177-180.

[20] Kato, Ikuko, Abraham MY Nomura, Grant N. Stemmermann, and Po-Huang Chyou. "A prospective study of gastric and duodenal ulcer and its relation to smoking, alcohol, and diet." American journal of epidemiology 135, no. 5 (1992): 521-530.

[21] Salih, Barik A., M. Fatih Abasiyanik, Nizamettin Bayyurt, and Ersan Sander. "H pylori infection and other risk factors associated with peptic ulcers in Turkish patients: a retrospective study." World Journal of Gastroenterology: WJG 13, no. 23 (2007): 3245.

[22] Levenstein, Susan. "Stress and peptic ulcer: life beyond helicobacter." Bmj 316, no. 7130 (1998): 538.

[23] Marucha, Phillip T., Janice K. Kiecolt-Glaser, and Mehrdad Favagehi. "Mucosal wound healing is impaired by examination stress." Psychosomatic medicine 60, no. 3 (1998): 362-365.

[24] NHS Choices. NHS. Accessed February 6, 2020. https://www.nhs.uk/conditions/stomach-ulcer/symptoms/.

[25] Hunt, R. H., Micheal Camilleri, S. E. Crowe, E. M. El-Omar, J. G. Fox, E. J. Kuipers, Peter Malfertheiner et al. "The stomach in health and disease." Gut 64, no. 10 (2015): 1650-1668.

[26] Rey, Johannes Wilhelm, Ralf Kiesslich, and Arthur Hoffman. "New aspects of modern endoscopy." World journal of gastrointestinal endoscopy 6, no. 8 (2014): 334.

[27] Levy, Stuart B. "The challenge of antibiotic resistance." Scientific American 278, no. 3 (1998): 46-53.

[28] Lesbros-Pantoflickova, Drahoslava, Irene Corthesy-Theulaz, and Andre L. Blum. "Helicobacter pylori and probiotics." The Journal of nutrition 137, no. 3 (2007): 812S-818S.

[29] De Francesco, Vincenzo, Floriana Giorgio, Cesare Hassan, Gianpiero Manes, Lucy Vannella, Carmine Panella, Enzo Ierardi, and Angelo Zullo. "Worldwide H. pylori antibiotic resistance: a systematic review." Journal of Gastrointestinal & Liver Diseases 19, no. 4 (2010).

[30] Pantoflickova, D., I. Corthesy-Theulaz, G. Dorta, M. Stolte, P. Isler, F. Rochat, M. Enslen, and A. L. Blum. "Favourable effect of regular intake of fermented milk containing Lactobacillus johnsonii on Helicobacter pylori associated gastritis." Alimentary pharmacology & therapeutics 18, no. 8 (2003): 805-813.

[31] Gotteland, Martín, O. Brunser, and S. Cruchet. "Systematic review: are probiotics useful in controlling gastric colonization by Helicobacter pylori?." Alimentary pharmacology & therapeutics 23, no. 8 (2006): 1077-1086.

[32] Jarosz, M., J. Dzieniszewski, E. Dabrowska-Ufniarz, M. Wartanowicz, S. Ziemlanski, and P. I. Reed. "Effects of high dose vitamin C treatment on Helicobacter pylori infection and total vitamin C concentration in gastric juice." European journal of cancer prevention: the official journal of the European Cancer Prevention Organisation (ECP) 7, no. 6 (1998): 449-454.

[33] Zhang, Hui-Min, Noriko Wakisaka, Osamu Maeda, and Tatsuo Yamamoto. "Vitamin C inhibits the growth of a bacterial risk factor for gastric carcinoma:

Helicobacter pylori." Cancer: Interdisciplinary International Journal of the American Cancer Society 80, no. 10 (1997): 1897-1903.

[34] González-Pérez, Antonio, and Luis A. García Rodríguez. "Upper gastrointestinal complications among users of paracetamol." Basic & clinical pharmacology & toxicology 98, no. 3 (2006): 297-303.

[35] Tarnawski, Andrzej S. "Cellular and molecular mechanisms of gastrointestinal ulcer healing." Digestive diseases and sciences 50, no. 1 (2005): S24-S33.

[36] Venturi, Sebastiano, and Mattia Venturi. "Iodine in evolution of salivary glands and in oral health." Nutrition and health 20, no. 2 (2009): 119-134.

[37] Wang, S-L., M. Milles, C-Y. Wu-Wang, G. Mardirossian, C. Leung, Amalia Slomiany, and B. L. Slomiany. "Effect of cigarette smoking on salivary epidermal growth factor (EGF) and EGF receptor in human buccal mucosa." Toxicology 75, no. 2 (1992): 145-157.

[38] Feitelson, Mark A., Alla Arzumanyan, Rob J. Kulathinal, Stacy W. Blain, Randall F. Holcombe, Jamal Mahajna, Maria Marino et al. "Sustained proliferation in cancer: Mechanisms and novel therapeutic targets." In Seminars in cancer biology, vol. 35, pp. S25-S54. Academic Press, 2015.

[39] Rivilis, J. E. F. F. R. E. Y., A. HOPE McARDLE, GEORGE K. Wlodek, and F. N. Gurd. "Effect of an elemental diet on gastric secretion." Annals of surgery 179, no. 2 (1974): 226.

[40] Mahmood, Asif, Anthony J. Fitzgerald, Tania Marchbank, Eleana Ntatsaki, Daniel Murray, Subrata Ghosh, and Raymond J. Playford. "Zinc carnosine, a health food supplement that stabilises small bowel integrity and stimulates gut repair processes." Gut 56, no. 2 (2007): 168-175.

[41] Taylor, Jennifer A., Benjamin P. Bratton, Sophie R. Sichel, Kris M. Blair, Holly M. Jacobs, Kristen E. DeMeester, Erkin Kuru et al. "Distinct cytoskeletal proteins define zones of enhanced cell wall synthesis in Helicobacter pylori." Elife 9 (2020): e52482.

[42] McGee, David J., Xiao-Hong Lu, and Elizabeth A. Disbrow. "Stomaching the possibility of a pathogenic role for Helicobacter pylori in Parkinson's disease." Journal of Parkinson's disease 8, no. 3 (2018): 367-374.

[43] Mulak, Agata, and Bruno Bonaz. "Brain-gut-microbiota axis in Parkinson's disease." World Journal of Gastroenterology: WJG 21, no. 37 (2015): 10609.

[44] Islami, Farhad, and Farin Kamangar. "Helicobacter pylori and esophageal cancer risk: a meta-analysis." Cancer prevention research 1, no. 5 (2008): 329-338.

[45] Rolig, Annah S., Cynthia Cech, Ethan Ahler, J. Elliot Carter, and Karen M. Ottemann. "The degree of Helicobacter pylori-triggered inflammation is manipulated by preinfection host microbiota." Infection and immunity 81, no. 5 (2013): 1382-1389.

[46] Fang, Boye, Huiying Liu, Shuyan Yang, Ruirui Xu, and Gengzhen Chen. "Effect of subjective and objective sleep quality on subsequent peptic ulcer recurrence in older adults." Journal of the American Geriatrics Society 67, no. 7 (2019): 1454-1460.

[47] Zullo, A., L. Gatta, V. De Francesco, Cesare Hassan, C. Ricci, V. Bernabucci, Mariateresa Cavina, E. N. Z. O. Ierardi, S. Morini, and D. Vaira. "High rate of Helicobacter pylori eradication with sequential therapy in elderly patients with peptic ulcer: a prospective controlled study." Alimentary pharmacology & therapeutics 21, no. 12 (2005): 1419-1424.

[49] Martínez-Maqueda, Daniel, Beatriz Miralles, Sonia De Pascual-Teresa, Inés Reverón, Rosario Muñoz, and Isidra Recio. "Food-derived peptides stimulate mucin secretion and gene expression in intestinal cells." Journal of agricultural and food chemistry 60, no. 35 (2012): 8600-8605.

[50] Shimotoyodome, Akira, Shinichi Meguro, Tadashi Hase, Ichiro Tokimitsu, and Takashi Sakata. "Short chain fatty acids but not lactate or succinate stimulate mucus release in the rat colon." Comparative Biochemistry and

Physiology Part A: Molecular & Integrative Physiology 125, no. 4 (2000): 525-531.

[51] Gaudier, E., A. Jarry, H. M. Blottiere, P. De Coppet, M. P. Buisine, J. P. Aubert, C. Laboisse, C. Cherbut, and C. Hoebler. "Butyrate specifically modulates MUC gene expression in intestinal epithelial goblet cells deprived of glucose." American Journal of Physiology-Gastrointestinal and Liver Physiology 287, no. 6 (2004): G1168-G1174.

[52] Bedford, Andrea, and Joshua Gong. "Implications of butyrate and its derivatives for gut health and animal production." Animal Nutrition 4, no. 2 (2018): 151-159.

[53] Candela, M. et al. Interaction of probiotic Lactobacillus and Bifidobacterium strains with human intestinal epithelial cells: adhesion properties, competition against enteropathogens and modulation of IL-8 production. Int. J. Food Microbiol. 125, 286–292 (2008).

[54] Sonnenburg, J. L. et al. Glycan foraging in vivo by an intestine-adapted bacterial symbiont. Science 307, 1955–1959 (2005).

[55] Holscher, H.D., 2017. Dietary fiber and prebiotics and the gastrointestinal microbiota. Gut microbes, 8(2), pp.172-184.

[56] Blanco, A., and G. Blanco. "Chapter 26-Biochemical Bases of Endocrinology (II) Hormones and Other Chemical Intermediates." Medical Biochemistry (2017): 573-644.

Printed in Great Britain
by Amazon

78129211R00071